WHEN LIFE

THROWS YOU

A CURVE

*One Girl's Triumph
Over Scoliosis*

ELIZABETH GOLDEN

Praise for *When Life Throws You a Curve*

An insightful, honest, and ultimately uplifting account of one girl's battle with scoliosis. Elizabeth Golden's book is filled with lessons about courage, acceptance, grace, and the importance of family and friends. An inspiration to us all.

—SUZY WELCH,
CO-AUTHOR OF THE INTERNATIONAL BESTSELLER – "WINNING"

Elizabeth describes how she didn't let scoliosis affect her outlook on life, just as I didn't let if affect mine. I hope that any girl facing an illness will read this book and be inspired.

—MARITZA CORREIA, OLYMPIC MEDALIST

Having dealt with my own scoliosis since I was a teenager, I applaud Elizabeth Golden for writing this insightful book and sharing her story with teenagers and their families.

—JOBETH WILLIAMS, FILM AND TELEVISION ACTRESS

Seen through the eyes of adolescence, Elizabeth describes her personal experience with spine surgery to correct scoliosis and expresses this with charm, candor and humor. At the same time, she does not sugarcoat the surgical procedure, the discomfort and the related anxieties. Significantly, she relates her own journey of personal growth with the acquisition of coping skills to deal with life's difficulties. It is this growth toward maturity and independence that makes her story so compelling. This is the book for anyone facing similar life challenges.

—DR. DENIS S. DRUMMOND,
EMERITUS CHIEF OF ORTHOPEDIC SURGERY,
THE CHILDREN'S HOSPITAL OF PHILADELPHIA

Patient networking, which this book helps facilitate, is critical to the education of patients and families about scoliosis. This book will result in more knowledgeable and honest discussions between the physician and patient, which is so important for a good treatment outcome.

—DR. RANDAL BETZ,
PAST PRESIDENT, SCOLIOSIS RESEARCH SOCIETY AND
CHIEF OF STAFF, SHRINERS HOSPITALS FOR CHILDREN – PHILADELPHIA

WHEN LIFE

THROWS YOU

A CURVE

One Girl's Triumph
Over Scoliosis

ELIZABETH GOLDEN

FIVE STAR PUBLICATIONS, INC.
CHANDLER, ARIZONA

WHEN LIFE THROWS YOU A CURVE

One Girl's Triumph Over Scoliosis

ELIZABETH GOLDEN

Linda F. Radke, President
Five Star Publications, Inc.
PO Box 6698
Chandler, AZ 85246-6698
480-940-8182

www.WhenLifeThrowsYouaCurve.com

Library of Congress Cataloging-in-Publication Data

Golden, Elizabeth, 1989-
  When life throws you a curve : one girl's triumph over scoliosis / by Elizabeth Golden.
    p. cm.
  ISBN-13: 978-1-58985-102-3
  ISBN-10: 1-58985-102-1
  1. Golden, Elizabeth, 1989---Health. 2. Scoliosis--Patients--United States--Biography. I. Title.
  RD771.S3G65 2007
  362.196'73--dc22

                    2007035955

Printed in the United States of America

Editor: Paul M. Howey
Cover Design: Maria Mann
Interior Layout: Maria Mann
Project Manager: Sue DeFabis

**In order to protect the privacy of individuals,
some of the names in this story have been changed.**

DEDICATION

I dedicate this book to my Grammy, without whom it could not have been written. It was her idea, her love and her genes that made it possible. She continues to help me grow and achieve my full potential.
I love her very much.

ACKNOWLEDGMENTS

Thank you Dr. Denis Drummond and all the amazing nurses and staff at the Children's Hospital of Philadelphia. I am a healthy girl who owes so much to all of you.

To all of my other caregivers who aided me before, during, and after my hospitalization, your work is incredibly honorable and the huge impact you have on lives like mine makes you akin to miracle workers.

I deeply appreciate both the energy and innovation with which my agent Ann Collette helped me in this entire process. More importantly, I would like to thank her for the wonderful bond we now share.

Thank you to Suzy Welch and her advice that I "write from the heart."

Thank you to Linda Radke, my publisher, for believing in me and caring about what I truly wanted.

To my editor, Paul Howey, thank you for accepting my work and keeping the language and story my own.

The first person to read my manuscript, Joanne Golden Ruchman, thank you for your interest in my story.

To Dr. Darryl Ford, thanks for supporting me throughout my operation and recovery.

Thank you to Rachel Malhotra, a fantastic English teacher who is largely responsible for helping me to learn how to write.

To Alice Davis, my favorite high school teacher, thank you for teaching me what it means to be a strong, proud, intellectual woman.

Thanks to my friends for being so much fun and for helping me during this time. To my campfriends Emily Krassen, Alex Lamm, Jill Reid, Molly Plotkin, and Ali Levi, you were there for me for the months after my operation and I will never forget your support. The fun I have had with you is unforgettable and I know we will be friends forever. To Rachael Wolf, Jessica Griffith, Amanda Davis, and Tory Pratt thanks for being amazing friends during my recovery. Jorie Dugan and Rebecca Garden thanks for reading my story and understanding me so well. You keep a smile on my face.

To my brother Robert, I will always love you very much and I know we will be close forever. Never stop being your unique and hilarious self.

My family was also deeply instrumental in the process of formulating this book. To Aunt Joanne who lived through this herself and helped me with both her advice and humor to make my experience so much better. Thank you to Aunt Sally for her amazing input, to Uncle Marc for his help with the overall picture, and to Aunt Leslie for her caring.

My grandparents have served to be excellent role models and supporters in this entire process. For always admiring who I am and encouraging me to stay true to that, thank you Grandfather, Nana, Papa, and Grammy.

Thanks to my parents for allowing me to tell my story with no limitations. I will never forget your love and support of me in everything we have gone through together. Thanks, Dad, for your help with the title and Mom for keeping me on schedule and helping to make this the best book that it could be. It is hard to imagine a better set of people and I am sure that I'm one of the luckiest kids on earth to have you two.

INTRODUCTION

Scoliosis can affect infants, children, and adults. It can affect boys as well as girls, but there is a much higher incidence of adolescent scoliosis among females. In fact, girls are seven times more likely than boys to develop a more severe curvature to their spines. There are an estimated one million teenagers suffering from scoliosis in the United States. To date, there is no known cure, although there are surgical procedures which can remedy some of the problems associated with scoliosis.

My name is Elizabeth Golden, and this is my story. I was diagnosed with scoliosis when I was 13 years old and in the seventh grade. The doctors told me my best option for a normal life was to undergo serious back surgery. With the support of my family and friends, I had the operation one year later. Following the surgery, my back was much better, although the doctors couldn't fully correct the curves in my spine.

I'm a typical teenager, but I'm truly nothing out of the ordinary. I want to share my story so that other kids with scoliosis (and their families and their friends, too) will know what it's like. My hope is my experience will provide you and your family with the strength and optimism to carry you through any medical challenge.

Chapter One

"We're ready for you now."

I looked up at the nurse, and then glanced around the surgery waiting room. I should have been freaking out, but I wasn't. I couldn't believe that getting my blood taken at the Red Cross a few months ago had left me sweating, shaking, and petrified. Yet now, when I should have been fainting with fear, I was calm and, as they say, cool as a cucumber.

Mom and Dad got up to go with me and the nurse; Grammy, and Aunt Joanne followed.

"I'm sorry, only your parents can go with you," said the nurse. My Grammy and Aunt Joanne seemed upset. After all, they'd been through this before, but not mom and dad. I knew the nurse was just doing her job. I have to admit that when I first saw her thin, pale face, I thought she looked intimidating. But then when she smiled, she looked nice, even trustworthy.

"You'll do fine," Grammy whispered, as she hugged me close. "Remember what happened to me. Having scoliosis has the power to bring out the best in you. Though I can't imagine you could possibly get any more perfect!" Usually this kind of cliché would have made me respond with a sarcastic remark. At this particular moment, however, I only had enough energy to nod.

"Just make sure they don't lose your underwear!" joked Aunt Joanne as she gave me a hug and kissed me. "They made me wear scratchy hospital underwear when mine went missing after my operation. Trust me, I'd rather have been stark naked!"

Believe me, underwear was the last thing on my mind. In fact, I wasn't thinking about much of anything. I felt almost numb. My parents, on the other hand, were trying really hard to hide how nervous they were. Mom's eyes were wide, and every so often she gave that fake cough she does when something makes her uncomfortable. Even my dad, who is a doctor himself, was clearly pretending not to worry. I thought maybe, if I acted like I wasn't nervous, they'd calm down. Since I already felt so weirdly detached, acting normal wasn't all that hard. I thought how ironic it was that I'd been about to hyperventilate the day before because of a huge history test. Now, here in the hospital where I had every right to be scared, I was fine.

I felt a sudden chill and began to shiver. I pulled my bluish-green hospital robe tighter around me as I got up from my chair. The robe wasn't much help in keeping me warm, as it was thin and made of paper. Still, tightening it made me less self-conscious about people seeing up the bottom of it. Other than the flimsy robe, the only thing I had on was the hospital ID bracelet fastened around my ankle. The bracelet looked like one of those cool plastic ones with holes all around it you get at amusement parks. I remembered the red one I'd gotten when my friends and I had gone to Six Flags. We decided they'd make great friendship bracelets, and I'd worn mine until Mom had made me take it off yesterday in preparation for the operation. I was sad to see it go, but it really was getting pretty gross. I asked the nurses to put the hospital bracelet on my wrist so I wouldn't miss the red one so much. But they said since I would be having IVs in my arms, it had to go on my ankle. Hearing about the IVs wasn't exactly comforting. At the moment, however, I was facing surgery so I didn't really care.

¤

Good laughs and fun times are two of my favorite things. Because I'm crazy about all my friends, naming my favorite people is much more difficult than naming my favorite sports (I like playing squash and tennis). My younger brother Robert is one of my best friends, though only on the days he decides to be normal and rejoin the human race. And then there are my parents, two people I love a lot. My family—my mom, my dad, my brother, and I—live in Philadelphia, Pennsylvania. Although at times we may seem slightly dysfunctional, we get along great. My second "family"—my friends—are amazing, and we are constantly laughing and acting crazy.

Another of my favorite pastimes is eating. I love nothing more than a big steak, mashed potatoes, and key lime pie for dessert. I love chocolate, too, but it makes my face break out, so I don't eat it that often. I don't want that to sound like I worry a lot about the way I look, because I'm really not like that. I have long, curly hair, but I don't do anything special with it everyday, and I rarely put on makeup. I do have something to confess though. I have been known to spend a really long time picking out what I'm going to wear. I have what I think is a style unique to me. I like to wear large, dangly earrings, jeans, and funky shirts.

My friends and family claim I can't sit still and I'll admit they're right. This has transferred over to how I live my life. I try to set high goals for myself, and I work hard in school. Overall, I just like to live my life to the fullest.

Like most kids, I've had many important experiences in my life. There's only been one, however, that had the power to change my life along with my body.

There are one million girls in the Unitede States who have scoliosis, a curvature of the spine. None of us thought it could happen to us. I knew that my aunt and grandmother had scoliosis when they were younger, and that it was hereditary. Still, until I was diagnosed, I never thought it would happen to me. Although I felt sorry for my aunt and grandmother and the others, I'll admit that I didn't really get what it meant to have scoliosis.

When I found out I had it, I immediately wanted to know what I was going to go through. I searched for other girls' stories everywhere, because I'm the kind of person who likes to know what she's getting into. I did research, talked to my doctors, and of course, to my Aunt Joanne and Grammy. I wanted to find out how it was back then for them, but also how it is now. I'd read how the technology has advanced so much it makes you feel lucky.

But in the surgery waiting room, as I looked around at the other pre-operative kids waiting with me, I forgot about everything I'd learned. All I could do was stare at the cheap linoleum floor, the bare walls, and bright lights. All my rational feelings flew right out of my head.

The nurse told me to lie down on one of the many stretchers that lined the long, windowless hallway. It almost looked like a parking lot with stretchers lined up next to each other in rows. After lying down, I remember being wheeled in front of a TV. *The Rugrats* was on (it's funny the little things one remembers during stressful times). Another nurse gave me a little cup of red syrup she said would make me fall asleep. I drank it and was delighted to find it tasted much better than the cough syrup I took at home. That stuff often made me gag. In just a few moments, a wave of sleepiness began to wash over me. I found myself subconsciously trying to fight the effects of the syrup, hoping somehow that if I stayed awake, I would have more control. I watched *The Rugrats* for a while and then looked at my parents.

Mom and Dad were standing on either side of my stretcher, each wearing the matching bracelets they had gotten, so that I couldn't leave the hospital without them. Mom was fiddling with hers now, a big fake smile stretched across her face. Having them by my side was a huge help. They started talking to me, trying to comfort me. I remember thinking that they looked like they needed me to comfort them. I felt sad because I didn't want them to worry, but I was tired and at the moment, had no energy to dwell on it. As tired as I was, I kept thinking that in just a short time, doctors were going to open up my back, place two rods and some hooks on my spine and then crank it as straight as it would go.

CHAPTER TWO

October 26, 2002, was a beautiful fall day. It was my Bat Mitzvah, and the time when I would become a Jewish woman. I felt great. At the service that morning, I had to read pages and pages of Hebrew and didn't make one mistake. I was bursting with self-confidence as everyone kept telling me I had done a great job, and my personal favorite compliment—how much they liked my sleeveless, baby blue silk dress. I was so happy as I sat at the table with all my closest friends, and watched the colored leaves drop to the ground.

We were in my backyard. Even though we live in the city of Philadelphia, our neighborhood feels more like the suburbs. Fall is beautiful here, which is why we decided to have the party outside. All the leaves were turning orange, yellow, and green, and the way the sun shone through the trees made it look like a beautiful painting moving in slow motion. Though I'd wanted a nighttime dinner and dance party, my mother said no. She had recently redone our house and I think she just wanted to show it off to all of her friends. So we had the luncheon at home. I was more than fine with that. In fact, it was really nice. The setting was calming and as a result it made the party more fun and less stressful for everyone.

The hors d'oeuvres were passed around in the house and then later, the main course was served in our front yard under a tent. In keeping with the party's autumn theme, the tablecloths had leaf print on them and each invitation had a real leaf pasted on the cover. A wooden dance floor was put next to the band and in front of the dozen tables so that women wouldn't get their high heels stuck in the grass. And as for my all-time favorite topic of food, it was scrumptious steak and salmon, delicious salads, and a huge dessert bar.

A great band played my pop and hip-hop music choices mixed in with enough of my mother's oldies to keep her and her friends happy. My friends and I got up and danced and everybody, including me, had a blast. It was so much fun, I didn't ever want it to end. I was enjoying sharing this day with my family and my best friends from overnight summer camp and school.

While my camp friends and I were considered the "cool group," my school friends and I were not. We weren't the opposite end of the spectrum, but we were certainly considered a level lower than the *real* cool group. In many ways, I thought my social status was perfect for both situations. At camp, I got to be around completely fun and self-confident people who always had juicy and interesting stories to tell about guys. At home, I had amazing, fun friends who didn't pressure me to do things I didn't want to do. I'm not saying everyone likes it that way. For me, however, it was the best of both worlds.

After I danced with some friends and a couple of old relatives, I started to look for Ali. She's my closest friend, and she'd made a photo album from all our good times and given it to me with a huge hug after the service was over. Ali was dancing over on the side of the dance floor. She'd apparently already made "enemies" with one of my camp friends, who asked me why I was even friends with her. I just laughed and said Ali was not the best at first impressions and could sometimes do and say inappropriate things. Though, to be truthful, that's what I liked so much about her. With Ali, you never knew what to expect and as a result, she's always a ton of fun. We laughed so much all of the time that my other friends sometimes got jealous of how close we were.

Ali is pretty in a self-confident way, though not like a model or anything. Our other friends say we look somewhat alike. In fact, our English teacher frequently confused us for one another. Both of us are medium-height and thin, with long brown hair, and dark brown eyes. We look so similar we were even able to make our school's only new eighth-grader think we were twins. As much as I love Ali, she's always had a competitive side, which has led her to be constantly surrounded by drama. In terms of our relationship, I hated fighting so when we had a conflict she usually had the upper hand. This was the only thing I didn't like about our friendship. Though the fights were rare they left me feeling horrible for days. I am really sensitive to insults and her ability to say the most hurtful thing possible, was hard for me to deal with.

I know all this stuff makes her sound like a bad person. In truth, Ali is great and she's the one person who really knows me the best. She's always thinking of ways to make me happy and of fun stuff for us to do. One of my favorite things about her is that she can make me laugh so hard tears run down my face. I hardly notice her flaws, because I like her good qualities so much.

I looked over at one of the tables and saw my squash coach, Julie. Seeing her reminded me that I had just found out I was ranked 33rd best girl squash player in the country in my age group. I work very hard at sports, because I'm not naturally gifted or anything. I take lessons twice a week and frequently play in clinics that are usually filled with younger, annoying boys. That part makes it not my favorite thing to do. I like sports though, because they are fun and help me stay in shape. Truth is, however, I'm not very competitive. I think that's held me back at times. Julie caught my eye and waved me over to her.

"Hey," she said. She was Australian, with an accent that sounded British to me. She has short, cropped blond hair and is in her forties, although she looks much younger. She is in much better shape than most people her age. Heck, she's in better shape than most people my age. "Are you having fun?" she asked.

"Yeah, this is a blast."

She smiled. "I heard about your national ranking. How does it feel? That's a big honor, you know."

"It feels really good. I was sort of surprised, to tell you the truth. I never thought that my work would actually pay off like that."

She smiled and said, "Well, you deserve it! You have so much potential. Just some more hard work and you'll be winning most of your matches, maybe a tournament or two." I was both surprised and excited by this last comment. I knew she wasn't just being nice. Because when Julie says something, she means it. "I'll let you go, I don't want to hold up the party girl."

"Thank you so much," I said, and I really meant it. "I'll see you on Tuesday for our lesson."

"You better come ready to run," she joked. "We need to burn off this delicious food." I waved goodbye, and I remember thinking that this day was the best ever.

Everything was better than great by the time Ali and some of my other friends got up to read a speech about their friendship with me. As embarrassing as all of this was, it was really flattering and the speeches were funny, too. I wasn't usually the most outgoing person in my group, but this was my day and somehow a new side of me was showing. Even my younger brother Robert, who at ten was three years younger than I, was being really sweet. He had been jealous earlier in the day about all the attention I was getting, but that had passed. He gave a speech about how much he loved me (that was a nice change from the "loser" I usually hear from him). Then he hugged me and even agreed to dance with me—when my mother requested it. He is sort of like my friends, but add in even more craziness. Robert is short with straight brown hair and puppy dog eyes. He has a very sarcastic sense of humor and loves to make fun of people. Plus, he wants to be an actor and loves attention, which explains why he was shaking his hips and shimmying across the dance floor at my party.

Next, my parents, Susan and Michael, each gave a speech. They are not the worst parents around, and I love them with their flaws. My mom has a high-powered job and it always seems like someone super-glued her cell phone to her face. My dad is a doctor and a genius. He is really nice and thoughtful, and is always the one who remembers to bring the things everyone else forgets, although it takes him two hours to get out of the house when we go anywhere. Both my mom and my dad have crazy hours at work. We usually eat dinner apart because they are so busy, but when we do get free time or when we go on our rare vacations, we have a good time. Everyone can tell how much we all love each other.

Near the end of the party, I went over to spend time with my grandparents. I am one of the lucky few who has all her grandparents alive and healthy. Nana and Papa are quiet and conservative, in contrast to Grammy and Grandfather who are extremely social and very active. I love them all very much and enjoyed hanging with them for a while during the party. Then I went over to see my Aunt Joanne.

"Hey girl!" she shouted. "What's happening? You were fantastic, and that dress is totally cool." My aunt is just that herself, so totally cool. She lives in New York City and is hilarious. She has shoulder length, dark brown hair and is pretty. She and my brother Robert have the same puppy dog eyes, except hers are blue. She prefers comfortable loose clothes and no makeup. Joanne works at MTV Networks, helping to launch the LOGO channel. She can get really preoccupied with her job and that sometimes means she misses family gatherings and forgets to call back family members.

"Thanks for coming, Aunt Joanne. When do I get to go to New York and check out your job at MTV? It's like the coolest thing ever. All my friends are so jealous and want me to bring back T-shirts for them. They're driving me crazy!"

"I can totally hook you guys up with T-shirts. Definitely come visit."

"Hey, I'm tying down the life of the party here," Aunt Joanne said. "Get out there before your old aunt bores you to death." We laughed and hugged goodbye.

I went over and sat down and began talking with my friends. I started thinking about my life. I can do that—talk and think at the same time. My dad calls it multitasking, but it's not like I can do the thing where you pat your head and rub your stomach. In terms of my life, everything was great, including the fact I'd managed to get all A's at my school,

Penn Charter. My school was exciting, the classes were interesting, and although the work at times could be hard, my teachers were absolutely amazing.

The party wound down and everyone told me how great it had been. Then we all said goodbye. This beautiful fall day had been absolutely ideal. Little did I know that three months from this perfect moment, my life would be turned upside down with news I'd never have expected.

CHAPTER THREE

I had been nagging my mother to schedule an appointment with my doctor for me to get a checkup, as I just wanted to get up to date with my shots. I love her to death, but my mother can't always be trusted to make my appointments. I understand why. Her job as a public relations executive takes almost all of her time and even when she manages to get off the cell and finish checking her e-mails, she's still consumed with thinking and strategizing about work. This causes her to forget some things related to our family, although to be fair, my dad isn't as involved with Robert and my schedules. At times, it's annoying to have such busy parents because I wish we had more time to hang out as a family. To be honest, I've sort of gotten used to it. Even though I sometimes think their priorities are mixed up, I know they love me.

I never wondered whether or not I was healthy. I guess I assumed that since I was young and active, I couldn't get really sick. As a result, doctor's appointments didn't make me nervous. In fact, I was happy to go after having to constantly nag and remind my mom to schedule them. That day in Dr. Lockman's waiting room was no different.

I was far from nervous, just watching the other people in the waiting room as I opened up the magazine that had been lying on the wooden table next to me. I flipped to a page displaying the ten cutest halter-tops of the season. Considering it was winter and my school's dress code barred sleeveless shirts, these fashion tips were not exactly helpful. Finally, my name was called and my mom and I were led to an examination room. Dr. Lockman came in with my chart and got started right away.

He was tall and thin with graying hair and eyes that twinkled. He was one of those adults who thinks he's hilarious and likes to crack jokes. Even though he had a loud booming voice, Dr. Lockman made me feel comfortable. My dad said he had a good reputation, so I trusted him. His examination room, where my mother and I were at the moment, was small and narrow with stenciled red and blue boats lining the top and bottom of the white walls. A brown, cushioned table was pushed up against the wall.

He did the usual. He checked my ears, eyes, mouth, etc. Everything was fine. So I was completely calm when he asked me to stand, bend over, and reach for the floor.

"Come over and look at this," he said to my mother. For once, she put her cell phone in her pocket and joined the doctor in the center of the room. I panicked a little when I heard my mother say, "That's strange. Isn't her spine … you know, curved?" She stopped talking and moved in for a closer look. "Her left shoulder-blade, is it higher than her right?" Her voice sounded worried, and I could tell that in a moment she was going to jump into her "keep your cool" mode, no matter what was happening. I had no idea what a curved spine meant. I just hoped it meant nothing at all.

Dr. Lockman's expression grew more serious and his voice got oddly soft. He said I had a minor curvature in my spine and that one shoulder blade was indeed higher than the other. "She'll need to see Dr. Ecker at Chestnut Hill Hospital. He's a scoliosis specialist there. At this point, it looks as though your condition is mild. It's important, however, that your progress be carefully monitored."

It didn't sink in at first, so I sort of sat there not knowing what to say. I wasn't prepared for any news like this. What did he mean by "at this point" my scoliosis was mild? Did that mean it could be worse in a few days? My heart fell. I got goose bumps and felt more nervous than I had when I played my fifth grade recorder solo in front of the entire class. As my fear grew, I started to get a funny feeling in my stomach. I didn't want to admit to myself what had just happened.

Another part of me started to get angry at Dr. Lockman. Even though I had really liked him just seconds before, I felt like this was somehow his fault. I mean, if I hadn't come in to see him, I wouldn't have had to worry about any of this. I was pretty much angry at the whole situation. After a few seconds though, my anger began to subside and I started to accept that this had nothing to with my doctor and that he was just trying to help me. I was left feeling sad and worried. I was scared, too. Really scared. All these doubts and a thousand questions were swirling around in my head.

¤

On the way home, my conflicting emotions became too much and I began to cry. My mom sighed and wiped away my tears ."Don't worry, honey," she whispered. That's all she said for a long time. I don't think she knew what to say. Besides, this was probably just as hard for her as it was for me. Finally she said, "Look, sweetie, we all have tough things that we have to face in our lives. This is yours. And I know you'll get through it perfectly." She reached over and took my hand. I glanced over to make sure her other hand was on the wheel. I didn't need a car crash to add to this day's horrible events!

"Scoliosis won't stop you from doing anything, whether you have to wear a brace or not," she added. "And if it doesn't progress, you'll be just fine. You have nothing to be scared about." I wanted desperately to believe her. But if she was telling me the truth, why was she crying? And what was this brace she was talking about? Right then, I didn't want to know.

When we got home, Mom suggested I call Grammy.

It was like déjà vu for Grammy, because she'd had scoliosis, too. I called her, but soon wished I hadn't because I soon found myself feeling the need to convince Grammy it wasn't her fault.

"Oh honey," she said to me sadly, "I can't believe I didn't notice it." At the very least, I should have been looking for it. I feel so responsible. It runs in families, so I just know you got it from my genes."

I tried to tell her it was okay, but she just kept talking.

"To be honest, since your mother didn't have scoliosis, I guess I didn't think you would get it either. Just know that change of any kind is sometimes hard to take, yet even if it seems bad, it can be a good thing. It ended up making me a better person."

I know she was trying to sound upbeat, but I could tell she was sad. I'm sure she just didn't want me to suffer. I'm her first grandchild, and she's forever thanking my Mom for giving her "this blessing, this ability to experience the joys and pleasures of having a wonderful grandchild."

She didn't say anything for a long time, and I found the silence kind of awkward. As I sat there holding the phone,

I could envision her closing her eyes, trying to think of the best thing to calm me down.

"Well, now there's an even more special bond between you, Aunt Joanne, and me," she said finally. "It can never be broken. We'll always be there for you with love and support. Believe me, we understand what you're going through."

Part of me truly doubted that she could understand how I was feeling at the moment. But still, it was nice to hear.

We talked for a few more minutes and then said goodbye. On an impulse, I dialed my Aunt Joanne's number at MTV. After going through a lot of assistants, I finally got her on the phone and told her what was going on. She tried to pretend it wasn't that big of a deal.

"I was in the sixth grade when a nurse in my elementary school made me bend over so she could examine my spine," she said. "I remember being glad, because the only other person who was singled out was a boy named Stephen. I thought he was really cute and I had a big crush on him. This was one of the few positives of getting scoliosis—having something in common with Stephen. At the time I thought it was a sign we were meant to be together, though it obviously wasn't. He didn't know I was alive and our relationship would have been hopeless."

She waited for me to stop laughing before continuing, "Aside from him, though, I didn't know anyone else who had scoliosis, except my mother. And up to that point, everyone thought she had gotten it from polio. But of course when I got it, they knew they were wrong because they'd since learned polio isn't hereditary."

Aunt Joanne promised to take the train to Philadelphia after work and tell me her whole story in person. That made me feel a lot better. I looked forward to more distractions, like her story about Stephen. Both Grammy and Aunt Joanne wanted me to feel like I was part of their "club." But quite frankly, it was a club I'd rather not join. Yet, I was happy to have them to talk to because I didn't know much about scoliosis. Not knowing made it scarier. I had no idea what was going to happen to me. Since I couldn't change the future, I decided I had to at least make an attempt to accept it. Of course, that stuff is always easier said than done.

All this worrying left me feeling exhausted, so I went up to my room to take a nap. About an hour later, I felt someone shaking me. It was my brother. "Mom told me about the scoliosis," said Robert. "Are you scared?"

For a little while at least, I had completely forgotten all about it. For the first time, I thought about whether I was scared. "I don't know," I finally managed.

"It will be okay. I hear when you're spine curves, you get a few inches shorter." He smiled and said, "maybe I'll finally be taller than you!" I laughed knowing that only Robert would think of this situation that way.

CHAPTER FOUR

I was so caught up in worrying about my diagnosis, I almost forgot about Dad. He still didn't know about it. He and I are really close, and I can always depend on him. He anchors our family down and keeps us sane. Even though as a doctor he has to work long hours, he always makes time for Robert and me. Sure enough, when he got home that evening from working at the hospital, my mother, acting all serious and upset, took him in another room and told him. After hearing the news, he came out to find me. He looked worried and told me he loved me and that he was sure I would be fine.

"Your whole family is going to be completely behind you in all of this. My feeling is, just be aware your condition exists, but don't worry about it. Scoliosis can be cured with a brace or an operation. Sometimes it's just a problem in terms of your appearance, and not a medical issue at all." He smiled. "You're a strong young woman. Nothing can hurt you." And then he hugged me. Out of all the people I'd talked to, he was the most comforting. He wasn't just my dad, he was a doctor. There was authority in what he said. At that moment at least, I was in a much better mood.

¤

That night, we all sat down for a family dinner (one of the few we had had in a while). We ate in our dining room that has seating for eight, a dark wooden floor, and a large, square, antique mirror on the wall. We live in a stone house with blue shutters that is at the end of a gravel driveway. It has four bedrooms. Robert's bedroom and mine are upstairs and my parents' bedroom is downstairs.

People say our house is warm and inviting, and I agree with them. The dining room, where we were now, was my favorite room. For dinner, we were having spaghetti and meatballs, with Caesar salad and Italian bread. I usually love this meal, tonight, however, I wasn't hungry. I ate anyway because I didn't want to worry my family. I even tried to keep up my end of the conversation. Robert and I talked about our teachers and school, while my mom talked about her interesting new client at work. Dad told us how happy he was we were all together. Still, I couldn't stop thinking about what effect my curved spine would have on my body. I didn't want to become a pretzel! As dinner was winding down, I asked, "Dad, how will scoliosis affect how I look?" I tried really hard to make it seem like the question was nothing special.

"You will be prettier than ever once this is over." He sounded confident, but it was hard to believe how having a big curve in my spine was going to improve my looks.

Mom had just brought out dessert of brownies and ice cream when the doorbell rang. It was Aunt Joanne. I had forgotten she'd offered to come over and tell me everything that night. "Hey guys, what's up? I missed you all tons." She hugged each one of us, giving Robert a high five. Robert and my aunt are really close, and they both have great senses of humor and love to laugh. She sat down and my Dad gave her a dish of ice cream. "Thanks, Michael," she said, before digging in. We all just made small talk while everyone ate their dessert. When we were done, Aunt Joanne came over and sat down next to me.

"Are you okay, sweetie? We're gonna have a long talk. I promise that you'll feel better by the end. Sound like fun? Your face seems to be saying no … now don't insult your fragile aunt," she said smiling. We started clearing our plates when all of a sudden Robert and my mom started to fight.

"It's Elizabeth's job, too, Mom," Robert insisted. "I'm not doing it without her."

"She's busy tonight. You can take out the trash alone."

"In your dreams! She always gets out of stuff." My brother's voice was rising with every word. "It's both of our jobs and so we are *both* going to take out the trash! You are so unfair. I'm not doing it without her!"

"Robert Golden! You are taking out the trash by yourself. Next time you're busy, Elizabeth will take it out for both of you." Mom was standing there with her hands on her hips.

"Fine, then I get her allowance for the week!" Mom just shook her head and turned away. My brother is an amazing negotiator and the only way to stop him is to end the conversation as quickly as possible. He gave her a few seconds to change her mind and when she didn't, he screamed, "Oh, shut up, Mom!"

"Robert, you do not say shut up to me. Now go to your room!"

He yelled something else at her as he ran up the stairs to his room. He made sure to slam the door with as much noise as possible. I felt bad because I think he was jealous of the attention I was getting from everyone, especially Aunt Joanne. The weird part was, there truly was nothing to be jealous about.

My parents, Aunt Joanne, and I went into the living room and sat down on the yellow sofa. It faces one of the room's three large windows that look out onto the trees, bushes, and flowers in our backyard. The living room is at the end of a long hall that runs the entire downstairs of our house. The room is comfortable enough, although we didn't usually sit there, except of course when something important happened. We spent most evenings in the kitchen. My news, however, seemed to qualify for the living room. I looked at Aunt Joanne with her ripped jeans and baggy sweater. She tucked her freshly blown out, shoulder-length hair behind her ears. She smiled at me, took a deep breath, and started her story.

Over the next several hours, Aunt Joanne told me how she'd been diagnosed with scoliosis when she was 12 years old. "You should be glad things have changed since then," she said. She described how she had to wear something called a Milwaukee brace. Which is basically an upper body cage made of steel and plastic that was designed to keep one's spine straight as their body continued to grow through adolescence. "I had to wear that awful contraption for 20 hours a day—*every* day."

"That had to have been terrible, Aunt Joanne," I said, trying hard not to imagine myself having to wear something like that.

"Oh, honey, you have no idea. Of course the braces today are a lot better and more advanced. But that thing had two vertical metal rods in back and one in the front that were attached at the bottom by a large piece of flesh-colored plastic that was molded around hips. The top was connected by a ring of steel to a plastic chin bar. And I was going into junior high! What would the other kids say?"

"What did they say?" I asked. I wanted to know. I, too, was worried about what my friends and the other kids would say. She told me everyone was very supportive, even throughout her operation and recovery, which had surprised her. I was at least somewhat encouraged by her story.

"Actually, I was lucky, because after my operation at Children's Hospital Boston, my surgeon, Dr. Hall, prescribed a fiberglass cast which was lighter and more waterproof than the older ones that most kids had to wear after surgery." Eventually, she said, the cast was removed. "I'm glad I went through all that, now that I look back on it," she said.

"You're kidding! Why would you say that?"

"No, I'm not kidding. I'm convinced it really has helped me throughout my entire life. At work, I sit higher and straighter than most people. With my stiff spinal column, I don't have a choice!" she joked. "Seriously though, I swear my erect posture adds credibility to whatever I have to say in meetings. The whole experience has made me a stronger person. I mean, nothing seemed impossible after I'd been through major back surgery. I wouldn't wish scoliosis on you or anyone, of course," she added. "But I know deep inside it's made me a stronger person."

CHAPTER FIVE

As I walked into Dr. Ecker's office, I couldn't get Aunt Joanne's story off my mind. Even though he specialized in scoliosis, I was still hoping it was all some big mistake, that I didn't really have scoliosis. I was afraid it would ruin my life and keep me from doing things I enjoyed.

A nurse called my name. I went with her into the room where she told me to put on a blue robe. Mom stayed with me while I put it on. We started laughing because I put it on backwards and was doing circles trying to tie the strings. When we finally got it on right, it was very big and thin and I felt naked. It made me think of that nightmare you have when your class sees you exposed in your underwear. This time, however, the doctor was part of the bad dream. I felt embarrassed and uncomfortable, so I tied the robe on as tightly as I could, but it still felt awkward and baggy. Somehow being forced to wear the robe made me realize just how real everything was. I was pacing back and forth when my dad came into the room.

I decided to sit on the doctor's examination table. I lifted myself up and in my nervous state, crumpled the paper on top of the table. It was loud and the sound, in addition to the cold table, made me shudder. I sat on the table, nervously swinging my legs back and forth. I finally understood that uneasy feeling my best friend Ali said she got every time she went to the doctor. It was terrible. I needed to get my mind off of scoliosis, so I tried to get my dad talking about his rounds at the hospital that morning. By the time Dr. Ecker came in, I had calmed down a little.

My first impression of Dr. Ecker was that he was old and fragile looking. He had gray hair, was short and hunched over (I wondered if he'd had scoliosis when he was younger and maybe that's why he'd chosen this specialty.) He seemed extraordinarily serious. I had never been to any kind of specialist before and didn't know what to expect. My heartbeat quickened. He shook my clammy hand and introduced himself. He looked smart and seemed experienced, so I relaxed a bit.

Dr. Ecker was a no-nonsense kind of doctor. He got right to the business of my scoliosis. I quickly decided he was okay and began to like him. He checked my back and pushed certain places to see if I had any tenderness. Nothing hurt that much except when he told me to roll down my socks and he brought out a needle. It wasn't even the type of needle they use for shots. Instead, it looked like a sewing needle. I wanted to say something sarcastic like we aren't in home economics class, but decided that wasn't a good idea. He pricked me in both ankles with the needle and I jumped. Apparently, jumping was good. He said if I hadn't felt it, it would have been a sign that I not only had scoliosis, but that it was more serious than most cases. It would have meant that I had defects in my nervous system rather than a hereditary gene that my relatives passed on to me. He could jab with the needle again if he was going to keep giving me good news like that!

Then he sent me to another room to get an x-ray. I'd never had one before, so I was really nervous. The nurse took me into a tiny room with a bed in the center and an expensive-looking camera hanging from the ceiling. The room was windowless, cold, and plain. There was something about that room that made me more worried and depressed. A medical technician told me to stand with my body pressed up against what looked like a dry-erase board. I expected to step behind the board and be able to see my skeleton through the other side, like I had seen on cartoons. It wasn't anything like that, however, and instead I just stood in three different directions while the technician took a picture from each angle.

She scared me because each time she would come back to replace the film, she had a blank look on her face. I couldn't read her expression at all. I wanted to know what she saw, but she was giving no hints whatsoever. She'd help me get into the correct pose, turn me to the side or to the front, and make me take a deep breath. Then she would leave me alone, feeling stupid and nervous. Each time she went outside, there I was standing all alone in a dark room, wearing an ugly robe, pressed up against a board and holding my breath. It would have seemed ridiculous if it hadn't been so scary. Once the third x-ray was completed, I was sent back to the examination room, where I waited with my parents for Dr. Ecker.

After a few minutes, he came in. "There are two curves in your spine, Elizabeth," he said. "One is small and the other is fairly big. I'm afraid you do have scoliosis." This news was not as hard to take as you might think, because I already knew that I had the curves. Then he told me I would have had only one curve, but my body had tried to even out the change by making a second one curving in the opposite direction. This explained why my head did not tilt off to one side. "Your scoliosis is cosmetic and won't be a threat unless the curves get worse." I let out a big sigh of relief. Unfortunately, he wasn't finished.

"And that has about a 70% chance of happening," he added.

Now I was more scared than ever. I had no control over whether my curve was going to get worse or not. My parents asked him what our options were.

"You can consider bracing," he said. "Bracing and exercises are the most common treatments for scoliosis. In my opinion, however, they don't guarantee results." Then he started talking to us about different medical studies he'd read. I ignored this part of the conversation and zoned out. I just wanted to know if I was going to be okay or not. I snapped back to reality in time to hear him finish what he was saying. He said the fact that my curve leaned irregularly to the left side could be a result of problems with my nerves, as some of those studies suggested. "Let's get an MRI, to be safe," he said. I'd heard of MRIs (magnetic resonance imaging machines) before.

From what I knew about them, I dreaded the idea. I'd been told they strapped you down in a small claustrophobic tube for a minimum of one hour and that you were not allowed to move a muscle. I remembered a scene from one of the all-time worst movies. It was about getting into the Navy and the tests you had to pass to be stationed on a submarine. One of the tests required you to be stuck in a small tank, half the size of a normal dishwasher, for hours. The man in the movie couldn't handle it and started banging on the tank for help. The door handle broke and he started having a panic attack. They finally pried him out, sweating, pale as a ghost and hardly able to breathe. It still gives me nightmares. I expected the MRI would also. I was scared, but my dad knew the right things to say. "Honey, an MRI is nothing. People get them all the time and they can't hurt you."

"Yeah, well, I'm still scared out of my mind. I might get claustrophobic."

"The tube isn't that small. Look, I send my patients to get them done when they need it. Do you think I would let them go if it weren't safe? Do you think I would let *you* go if it weren't safe?"

"I guess not. But either you or mom have to come with me though."

"I promise both of us will be there."

¤

A few weeks after my meeting with Dr. Ecker, I went to get an MRI at Children's Hospital in Philadelphia. The great thing was, I was allowed to bring a movie with me. When I watch television or a movie, I usually block everything else completely out. Whenever I'm talking to Ali on the phone, even if we're having a deep conversation, the second I walk by a TV, I go silent and forget everything else but the show. I don't drop the phone or anything, though that's probably because my body freezes into position. Ali gets really frustrated, and it's actually sort of funny. It doesn't even have to be a good show. I've noticed that Robert and Dad do the same thing, so maybe it runs in the family. Usually this isn't a good thing, because no one can get my attention, but for the MRI it could be a huge help. We stopped at the video store and rented *The Princess Diaries*, one of my favorite movies. It was very hard to choose a movie, because I wasn't supposed to move during the MRI. If the movie was scary or funny, I might jump or laugh, and then they'd have to start the MRI all over. Since I'd already seen *The Princess Diaries* a bunch of times, I figured nothing in it would be a surprise to me, except maybe how good it was the tenth time around.

The day of the MRI, I wasn't allowed to eat or drink any-thing except for apple juice. By the time we got there, I was starving. At lunch at school that day, a girl at another table was being nice and handing out small slivers of mango. Ev-eryone was taking a piece and eating. I wanted to be cool and, of course, I like food, so I took a slice, put it in my mouth, and swallowed. All of the sudden, alarms went off in my head. It was like the mango had pushed some kind of panic but-ton. Part of me was angry at myself for not telling Ali about the MRI, because she sat next to me at lunch and she might have been able to stop me. I didn't want to call my parents, because I was afraid they would get mad at me for forgetting. When they picked me up early from school to go to the MRI, I decided to tell them. They were kind of upset, especially my mom, because I'm forgetful a lot and it seems to always mess things up. Finally though, my dad said, "that's okay, things will work out." This whole problem made me completely forget how nervous I was about getting the MRI.

When we got to the hospital, I was told that I could still have the MRI but, because of the mango, I couldn't be se-dated or given an IV to make me go to sleep. Personally, not getting a huge, annoying needle in my arm was not exactly bad news, although I did realize that it would be hard to con-trol myself now that I would be awake and have to lie still for such a long period of time. Now I was really depending on the movie to make me chill out.

By the time we got to the clinic for the MRI, I was no longer scared. It was one of those times when I can't ex-plain why I felt so calm. I happened to notice a little boy about three years old sitting to my left in the waiting room. I watched as he was being sedated. They'd stuck a big IV needle in his hand that I hadn't noticed at first. But when I did, I got queasy. Needles and getting injections are not my favorite things. I didn't want to be mean, so I pretended I needed a tissue and got up. When I came back, I sat on the other side of my parents, away from the boy and his needle. I decided that if anyone told me they were going to get an MRI, I'd tell them to eat a mango. I was smiling at my own joke when they called me into an exam room.

The first thing the nurse told me to do was to get changed into another one of those "lovely blue robes," as my mother now called them. My parents were then asked to remove their phones, credit cards, and other random things. "The MRI machine might break them," the nurse said. I laughed when I saw Mom hurriedly carrying her cell to safety.

If the MRI could break cell phones, what could it do to me? I began to worry what would happen if I moved. I was scared to death I'd mess up the MRI and have to do it over. I was more worried about that than the actual MRI itself. As we walked by a window to one of the MRI rooms, the nurse pointed out a baby in one of the machines. The MRI machine was like a chute, longer and lighter than my war movie had led me to envision, yet still small and creepy enough to make me nervous. The lights inside of the tube illuminated the baby in an eerie way. Somehow I couldn't imagine myself lying in there, looking into the light, and not moving for hours. The baby's father sat in a rocking chair to the side in the room, looking understandably worried. I felt so sorry for him. All of a sudden, I felt really sorry for my parents, too. Of course, I hadn't meant to, but I knew I was causing them and others so much stress and heartache.

As we walked down the hall to my room, I grabbed my

mother's hand. That gave me the extra strength I needed. I was ready to take on the challenge. Once in the room, the nurse told me they were going to do what she called "three sequences" on my upper, middle, and lower back. I laid down and she gave me a pair of heavy, prism glasses so I could see the movie while I lay flat on my back. Next, she placed a pillow under my head and put earphones on me that sealed out the machine's noise but still allowed me to hear the movie. (My mother told me later she wasn't given earplugs and that when she was sitting in the room with me, it sounded like someone was using a jackhammer by her head.) The nurse gave me a squeeze ball so I could call her in case I needed anything. It just looked like a dog's chew toy, but holding it made me feel better and helped me remember that I was not alone. The nurse warned me that I would have to wait till the end of a sequence for them to respond to my requests. I was beginning to regret eating that mango. I now wished I could be put to sleep. She told me I couldn't fall asleep on my own because I might move. I froze every muscle in my body and heard the movie starting. I tried to see the movie through the prism glasses, but the images were all blurry. I squeezed the ball and a voice called out, "Are you okay?"

I told them what was wrong, that the movie was all messed up. A nurse came in and fixed it. She was very nice, but I felt guilty that I had already interrupted the whole process before we'd even gotten started. The machine started to rumble again and I tried to lie perfectly still. Thankfully, *The Princess Diaries* movie made the time go by very quickly. My mind felt totally clear. I also felt almost as if I was on Jupiter and the intense force of the planet's gravity was pinning me down. It was a weird sensation.

About halfway through, I got an itch on my arm. All I could think about was the itch. I struggled with it silently because I knew I couldn't move until the MRI sequence was finished. The itch became unbearable, almost painful. It started to feel like I'd broken my arm right down the center. I even stopped concentrating on the movie as the itch began to engulf my whole body. I tried to think about something else—*anything* else. I wanted to get done as quickly as possible, so I didn't want to squeeze the ball again. Although the nurse had been nice when I called her before, I had sensed a bit of annoyance and didn't want to get her mad. She had the power to make me stay for extra hours if she wanted. When the sequence was over, I immediately started scratching my arm. It was one of the most amazing sensations I'd ever experienced.

The nurse used a microphone to talk to me after every sequence to see how I was doing. I told her I was doing fine. At one point, however, while I was watching the movie, the grandmother in the story walked across the screen, slumping as if to imitate her granddaughter. It was hard not to laugh at that. I was proud of myself because I only let one little "ha" slip out. It turned out though that this one little "ha" was enough to require starting the entire sequence over. Even though I was afraid the nurses were angry with me, I knew inside it was an honest mistake. As time went on, I felt heavier and heavier like I must have weighed three hundred pounds. It was as though a sumo wrestler was sitting on me, pinning me down.

After one-and-a-half hours of successful stillness, I was finally done. When they pulled me out of the tube, the nurse and my mother had to help me sit up. It was the oddest feeling, like I'd lost two hundred pounds in that one split second. When I stood up, my legs gave out, and I would have fallen flat on my face if my mother and the nurse hadn't been holding onto me.

Afterwards, as a reward, my family took me to the White Dog Café for dinner. "I'm extremely proud of you," Mom said to me. "You've proven how strong a person you are." That was really nice to hear. More importantly, I had surprised myself, and that felt even better.

¤

Dr. Drummond was the second scoliosis doctor I met. My dad had heard about him from other doctors he worked with at The Hospital of the University of Pennsylvania. Dr. Drummond had a reputation for being a fantastic surgeon, and Dad said he was nationally known. I walked into Dr. Drummond's waiting room with my parents, and while they filled out some forms, I picked up a magazine and stared blankly at the pages. The office was childish, designed to look like a jungle with pictures of wild animals on the walls.

"Elizabeth Golden," a nurse announced. I got up absent-mindedly and started following her and my parents to the examination room. Halfway there, I realized I was still clutching the magazine, and I ran back to leave it in the waiting room. When I entered the examination room and sat down, I began thinking about how the distraction of having scoliosis had made me even more forgetful than I usually was.

My parents and I talked and joked. It didn't really matter what we talked about or what the jokes were. We were just helping each other relax. Dad stepped out of the room while I put on yet another of those blue robes I hated. It was scary to think that I was beginning to wear these ugly things almost as often I wore my own clothes. I felt exposed, yet after Dr. Drummond came in with my dad, I didn't think about it anymore.

My mom had brought my x-rays from Dr. Ecker's office, along with the results from my MRI. Dr. Ecker had told me my upper curve had a 70 percent chance of progressing, and the curve couldn't be stopped by a brace or anything else. Instead of saying the same thing, however, Dr. Drummond said he believed the curve had only a 30 percent chance of progressing and that corrective methods could be effective. That, of course, made me like Dr. Drummond right from the start. In addition, Dr. Drummond said he was going to do everything he could to prevent me from having an operation.

I was confused—and not just a little upset—by the fact the two assessments were so different. I hated not knowing what would happen to me. Then Dr. Drummond suggested I consider wearing a brace. Now I was really upset, and my eyes filled with tears. My mom got upset, too, even though she tried not to show it. I was afraid the brace would ruin my life, and I worried about what Ali and my other friends would think of me. That was the exact moment when any hope that I might not really have scoliosis slipped away. I felt like a light had turned off inside of me. Dr. Drummond continued talking and explaining things, but I'd stopped listening. I was devastated, more so than I had ever been in my life.

Before he left, Dr. Drummond said I would probably have to consider a Milwaukee brace because of my unique high curve. That was the same horrible contraption Aunt Joanne had told me about! Because my curve was unusual, the more modern braces wouldn't be effective. Dr. Drummond said I'd only be able to take it off for sports and showers. He showed me a picture of one. If I'd been upset before, I was now completely miserable. Just as Aunt Joanne had described it, the Milwaukee brace was ugly, big and very noticeable. The brace was obvious and embarrassing. It had a bar that came up around the neck. The bar was hooked to what Dr. Drummond admitted was "an uncomfortable shoulder sling." If all this weren't just horrible enough, he concluded by saying there was a high likelihood that, in the end, the bracing might not work. Nothing seemed to be going my way. I remembered Aunt Joanne telling me that her brace hadn't worked, and that they ended up operating on her anyway.

Dr. Drummond looked at me and said, "Elizabeth, don't get upset prematurely. This may not have to happen if later we find your curve has not progressed." He smiled and asked me to come back in four to six months.

Mom, Dad, and I talked about the appointment all the way home. That kind of surprised me, because usually we avoid touchy subjects. I guess this was just too big a problem to ignore. Eventually, I started to feel just a little bit better. I knew I would find a way to make things work out. Besides, what choice did I have?

Chapter Six

A few days after my MRI, I found out that Sara, a girl in ninth grade at my school, had scoliosis, too. She'd had the operation two years ago. It turns out my mother had called the director of my middle school that day and informed him about my "situation." In that conversation, he told Mom about a girl named Sara who had scoliosis. He called and asked her if she would talk to me and she said yes. He gave me her number.

Sara was really nice and a big help. Ali's sister was her friend, so we vaguely knew each other. At first I didn't want to call her because I thought it might be awkward talking about something so personal with someone I had never met before. But my mom said that discussing it with someone my age would be really helpful and since I trusted her advice I made the call.

Sara told me everything that had happened to her, and how everything had turned out okay. She offered to answer my questions at any time. I liked talking to her not just because she was comforting, but also because she didn't try to conceal anything. I didn't want to be sheltered. She told me that scoliosis, of course, wasn't always fun, but that it had simply become part of her life. She let me know there was a bunch of other kids in my school who had scoliosis. I couldn't believe I'd gone from not knowing what the word meant to being deeply immersed in the world of scoliosis.

That weekend, Ali and I met up at our favorite pizza restaurant. The pizzas are delicious and a lot of kids hang out there because it's affordable and fun. It has huge ovens, nice staff, and tons of booths. The atmosphere is great, with dim lighting and lots of noise. Ali and I were seated at a corner booth and given menus. While we were looking them over I asked, "So what are your plans for the rest of the weekend?"

"Just homework. My parents want a family night." She paused, "So basically I have no plans, unless you consider watching *Hello, Dolly!* with your family, a 'plan.' With my family, it's more of a chore." It was weird the way Ali talked about her family. Sure, they spent a lot of time together; but what was so bad about that? I was sure she wouldn't want to be me, who barely had family time at all.

We decided to order and our waiter came over. He was a tall guy with shoulder-length straight hair and a goatee, and I could tell Ali was going to flirt. I ordered first, asking for a slice of cheese pizza and a salad. Ali ordered next, although in the beginning she just sat there silently, crushing on the waiter. I laughed and kicked her under the table. Luckily, it was enough to snap her out of her "love trance" so she could ask for a slice of veggie pizza. She kept staring at him as he walked away. "He's cute," she sighed dreamily. "He looks like Brad Pitt, don't you think?" Personally, I thought he was average looking. He resembled Brad Pitt about as much as I resembled Yoda from *Star Wars*. After Ali had had enough time to get over the waiter, we talked about random stuff until the salad came. It was huge. It looked like they had gone to a gigantic farm and decided to put all of the lettuce in one bowl and surprise! When the waitress (I think Ali had scared the waiter off) delivered it and could hardly lift the thing, Ali and I started cracking up.

"We clearly must look too thin as far as the chef is concerned," I said sarcastically. Ali laughed and took the salad tongs. I could tell she was still a little upset that the waiter hadn't come back. In anger, she squeezed the tongs together before she put them in the salad, stuck them in deep, and was about to take salad when she realized she was holding them closed. When she released her grip and the tongs snapped open, salad flew absolutely everywhere and before we knew it, we were covered in greens. We both started laughing until tears were streaming down our faces. This moment was going to go down in the history of our friendship. If we didn't already look stupid enough covered in lettuce, now we were convulsing with laughter. We picked off the greens, wiped the tears off our faces, and went to the bathroom to wash off. "We are so not coordinated," she joked. When we were done, we went back and realized the waitress had been nice enough to clean off our table, including the salad!

"They probably wanted to make sure we didn't have any more ammunition," I said. "I've never thought of veggies as weapons, but anything is possible." We laughed and sat down again. The pizza came and while we ate, we reminisced and talked about all kinds of stuff. I finally felt like it was a good time to bring up my back. I wanted to talk to Ali about it because it was the main thing going on in my life at that moment. I hadn't told her before because part of me was hoping I might not actually have it. "So I need to tell you something. I have scoliosis. Basically my spine is curved."

"Really? Is that bad?" She looked worried, which I didn't want her to be, but I needed to continue.

"I have two curves that could either be a problem or not. We don't know for sure yet. If they keep getting worse, then it's a big problem because it could hurt my breathing or make me unable to have kids." She gasped. "Don't worry though," I assured her, "there are ways to stop it from getting that bad, like bracing and exercises. And if it does get worse, the doctor said I can have an operation. On the other hand, if it doesn't get worse, then I'm totally okay!" I surprised myself at how confident I sounded. I'd been able to comfort myself more than I had been comforted by everyone else put together.

"I'm so sorry, Elizabeth."

"This whole thing is crazy. I'm sorry too, Ali." I looked at my best friend and sighed. I definitely agreed with her that it was upsetting, because it was by far the worst thing I had ever experienced. We talked for a while longer and then paid the cashier and went our separate ways. The whole way home, I thought about my back. I wondered if Ali would still be my friend and if we would still have good times like today if I got disfigured. After tonight, I was pretty sure she'd always be my best friend.

¤

Long before this thing with my back happened, my parents had hired a personal trainer to supervise their exercise program at home. Since my doctors said exercise might be helpful in remedying my condition, I started joining my parents and the trainer for an hour each week in our gym in the basement. We worked with free weights, stretched, and used weightlifting machines. I'm not positive whether this did anything or not. I do know, however, that exercise made me stronger and more prepared for a possible operation. Most times, all this exercising was boring and hard. But it did have its upside. I got to spend time with my normally busy parents, and that was great.

That spring, I went to a chiropractor with my mom and my brother. Mom thought a chiropractor might be able to help my back, and Robert came along because my mom didn't have time to drop him off at home after school. He didn't care. He loves adventures and drama, and that's just what he thought a visit to the chiropractor would be.

We showed up at a small white building. It looked like a house that had been converted into an office. After my mother filled out a consent form, we were led into a small room with a television in it. I watched a movie promoting chiropractics. In the video, there were people talking about their successes with chiropractors. At first, their stories made me less nervous, but after the tenth story, the miracles were getting harder to believe and it made me second-guess what I was about to do.

My chiropractor was a tiny, mousy woman who was wearing a huge, sparkling cross around her neck. It was covered in fake diamonds, like it had been some rapper's "ice." Frankly, she looked ridiculous and strange. She sat me down and told my brother and mother to sit on chairs in the corner of the room. She talked to us for a few minutes, telling us this was a new job and that she had come from another state after her husband died. I didn't fully trust her and was suspicious of her reason for leaving home. I mean, what if she was a criminal? I imagined her having to run from the law because she stole Tupac's necklace or even worse, had killed her husband. Okay, I knew my theories were ridiculous and not so nice; but still, they made me trust her even less. She then took me over to a machine and had me sit on the stool in front of it. It was metal and looked ancient and clunky. It was shaped like a podium, and on the part where you would put your hands during a speech there was a computer screen. The screen had a graph on it that was part of a computer program. The woman explained that she was going to measure the heat in my back, heat generated by muscle activity which in turn would tell her what areas in my back needed stress relief. She had two little things that looked like inkpads that she moved up and down my spine. This supposedly showed the stress level of my whole back. I'm sorry, but it seemed like voodoo to me, especially because of all the "look at the colors on the screen, they will tell all" stuff. If my back was okay, the machine lights would turn green, she explained. If my back was stressed in places, then it would turn red. My whole spine ended up being red. Surprise, surprise. I couldn't catch a break.

She then had me lie down on the table and immediately started cracking my neck and arms with her hands. She continued to do more cracking, and it hurt. I was wondering why it didn't feel better, and she told me that eventually, with more treatments, my back would crack more easily. At this point, I looked over at my brother and my mom sitting in the corner of the room. They were flinching and jumping at every crack. Robert looked especially uncomfortable and kept whispering to my mother, loud enough for me to hear, "This is ridiculous." I was pretty sure I also heard him say, "That lady is a psycho killer."

The pain grew worse as she cracked her way up my neck. The cracking noises kept getting louder and louder. I guess I must have jumped or tensed up, because she told me to relax. She tried explaining that the cracking just sounded louder when it was closer to my ears. When she finally noticed that my family was going berserk, she said, "Oh, don't worry. I'm just relieving the stress on her muscles." My little brother, being the person he is, just had to respond. "It's just that we hate cracking in our family," he said with a straight face.

"OOH, ooh, ooh," she admonished. "Do not use the cracking word!" Robert rolled his eyes. Finally, she said I was done and I sat up. I was feeling a little nauseous, but the feeling soon passed. As we left, Robert whispered to me, "Tell that lady I am not two years old and that cracking is a hoax." And for once, I thought my brother had a point.

"We were scared for your life each time she cracked your spine," he said. "She probably had to leave the state because she killed her husband." I smiled because I had thought the same thing. My mother shushed him, but I knew she had not liked it either. After a pause she said, "how ironic that we hate when people crack their knuckles and we still end up at a chiropractor."

I turned to her and said, "ooh, ooh, mom. Don't say the cracking word." We all started laughing and I was happy that we had at least gotten a joke out of something that was clearly a failure.

After we stopped laughing I started to think about what had actually happened and got upset. Going to the chiropractor was not going to work as far as I was concerned, and that knowledge left me feeling more discouraged than ever.

My family's personal trainer recommended that I go to her friend who was a massage therapist. She believed that if you massaged the spine, it might straighten the curve. My family and I were still willing to try more alternative healing, so we decided to give it a shot. The appointment sort of caught me by surprise, though. We'd talked for a month about trying it and nothing had happened. Then one afternoon, Mom told me she had gotten an appointment with the massage therapist due to a last minute cancellation. We jumped in the car and off we went.

I have to admit, I was excited because I love massages. They feel so good, especially because I have so many knots in my back. At camp, my friends and I used to get in a circle and do a massage chain. This massage, however, would be very different, because now scoliosis was involved. I had no idea how this massage was supposed to fix my curve. Robert tagged along again for the same reason as last time.

We drove about 30 minutes to a residential neighborhood where all the houses looked the same: tan stucco, black shutters, short driveways. We ended up getting terribly lost and it got much later and darker before we finally found the house. The woman worked out of her home. That part was all right, but then she said to follow her out to the garage. Okay, now I was getting worried.

She was dressed in casual clothing and was a tad overweight, short, and looked like she was in her fifties. We followed her through her garage, which was full of bright beach toys and power tools. Robert kept on giving me this "OH, MY GOD!" look, which made me laugh out loud. But honestly, I was getting more nervous at the same time. Mom, who was walking ahead of us, looked equally worried about the woman's bizarre home office. We then walked through the garage to a wood-paneled room that had a padded table in the center and a chair on either side of the table.

She asked me about my scoliosis and about the methods I'd tried so far. Then she told me to stand up and demonstrate proper posture. I was definitely thinking she needed to focus on fixing my curve, not my posture. To my surprise, she pulled my mother over and told Mom that *she* had the worst posture she had ever seen. My mother was not amused. I guess the woman was hoping to get another patient to work on. After I changed into a robe, which of course I now despised, the "garage masseuse" came back into the room. I did a double take when I saw she was wearing a tool belt. But instead of tools, there were oil bottles in each little pouch. She turned on some music that sounded like waves crashing on a beach. I'm sure this was supposed to calm me down, but instead it just made me more nervous. The whole situation was freaking me out. She put oil on her hands and started massaging my back while I read the signs she had on her walls: "Life Is Worth Living" and "Peace is the Answer." I began wondering if she was both crazy *and* strange. *Great, just what I needed*, I thought. *Another kook to screw with my back.*

As she massaged my back with hot oil, she talked about her "successes." According to her, a woman had come to her distressed because she was shaped like a pretzel and unable to walk. The woman had tried many other methods and none had worked. This massage therapist worked on her hip and said the patient got better. Eventually, the woman could walk just fine. "She was a knot, all I had to do was untie her," she said. Okay, so maybe the story was true. I tried to convince myself she wasn't a quack. Still, part of me wondered if she was just playing it up and trying to get a new steady customer. Her stories were interesting enough, but my family and I wanted results.

My mom and brother kept on giving me strange looks as the woman continued talking. She told me about nutrition and what I should eat to stay healthy. I wanted to tell her that she should be focusing on the problem at hand, but I was afraid she would hurt my back if she got annoyed. I mean, she was already pushing down really hard. The woman started to talk about her life and then asked me about mine. I told her my age, though I didn't want to talk to her. I was afraid that the distraction would make it harder for her to do her job. Besides, I was having trouble talking because it was hard to breathe. My back started hurting a lot, but I kept telling myself I was willing to endure the pain if this method worked.

As I've mentioned, due to the curve in my back, one of my shoulder blades was higher than the other, and a lot of what she did was put intense pressure on that shoulder blade. For about ten minutes, she wasn't even massaging, just putting her weight on one shoulder blade. I couldn't see what skill was involved in pushing and how it would help. I mean, why did I need to come here for this when I knew Robert could have "pushed" just as well? When she told me she was going to loosen my joints, I had a flashback to the chiropractor. The only difference was the lack of loud cracking sounds. Surprisingly though, I found the massage to be more painful.

When she finally said she was done, I got dressed quickly and we left. As you might have guessed, this method had absolutely no effect on my curve. On our way home, my brother and my mom talked about how appalled they were by the woman. "We were basically in her *garage*," said Robert, "right next to her sleds and stuff." The massage method was definitely ruled out. My options seemed to be dwindling.

CHAPTER SEVEN

My next appointment with Dr. Drummond was scheduled three months later for March. My dad had asked for an appointment then, instead of the recommended four to six months, because if I did need an operation, an appointment in March would give me enough time to recover so I could still go to summer camp. For those next three months, my family, friends and I went about our lives and tried to do everything other than think about scoliosis.

I went to school and focused on working hard. Despite this, I got my first C. It was on a grammar test in English. Grammar and I do not mix well. It wasn't even hard stuff, but I was distracted. Ali got an A, even though I had studied with her. "How did you get a C?" she asked. "That's not like you." She could tell I was upset. "You'll do well on everything else, and your grades will be fine," she said trying to console me. "Hey, it's not like middle school matters or something."

I managed a weak smile and decided to study all weekend for the test on *Romeo and Juliet*. I ended up getting an A on that one. It definitely made me feel better about everything, because I couldn't deal with worrying about school and my back at the same time.

Not everything was about school. Actually, besides English, my classes had gotten easier as the year went on. I had a lot of free time, most of which I spent with my friends. Ali and I hung at each other's houses, but our parents got fed up at us being around so much, so we were mostly at other people's houses. Occasionally, we went to the movies, too.

Besides spending time with my friends, I also hung out with my family. We started to have family dinners more often and, for whatever reason, my mom seemed to be working less. It was like my family knew something was coming and we were banding together before the crash. We talked a lot, and I learned that my mom and dad's jobs weren't as boring as I'd thought. Dad's job has a lot of potential for excitement. If someone has a sudden health emergency, they call him in to fix it. He's a surgeon and from what my mom said, is very good at his job and widely respected. Of course, being a doctor has its downside, too. Occasionally, some people are beyond saving. Others sometimes decide not to be operated on, even if it means they'll die without the operation, and might even have a good chance of getting better. When he told me all that, I decided I never wanted to be a surgeon.

Mom's job is pretty much the opposite of my dad's, or at least it seems that way to me. She spends a lot of time in the office, making calls and e-mailing. She's an executive at a public relations firm. But until we did all this talking, I had no idea about all the research, preparation, and strategizing she has to do for her clients. She also told me some wild stories about her high school and college years. I couldn't believe my mom could be so much fun! I learned that she'd thrown her birthday cake out the dorm window on one occasion and had gone streaking through the boy's dormitory with her friends on another!

I also got to know more about my brother. Apparently, he was being chased around by tons of girls. From what I had heard, he was the most popular guy in his grade, and it seemed to be true, as our phone was constantly ringing. "Hello, is Robert there?" a young squeaky female voice would say. After

a while, it got annoying and I began to recognize the most fre-
quent numbers on our caller ID. When it would ring, I would
let it go, telling myself that either Robert would get it himself,
or the girl could wait to talk to him the next day at school.

¤

When the time finally came for my next checkup, my life
had been going so well I felt certain I was going to get good
news. Everything else was so perfect that it seemed nothing
could mess it up. My dad was standing outside Children's
Hospital waiting for us, because we were late. My mom and I
roared up to the front of the hospital and I threw open the door
and jumped out of the car. Dad and I ran upstairs to the waiting room. We filled out some forms and then they sent me over
to get an x-ray. On our way to get the x-ray, I saw a boy waiting
in the next room. I wondered if he had butterflies like I did.

This time, they took several pictures—one x-ray from the
front, one from the side, and two others where I was asked
to lie down on a table and bend to one side as far as I could.
After they were finished, I waited outside for them to be developed. When they were done, my dad and I took them and
went back over to the doctor's waiting room where my mom
finally joined us. Within a few minutes, the three of us were
walking rather nervously down the hall to the exam room.

I changed into the hated robe. I wasn't nervous about it
anymore. The robe had become a signal that I was to switch
into scoliosis mode. It was like my alter ego. When I was
in the robe, I was dealing with my back. When I put on my
regular clothes and left the doctor's office, I was back to my
normal life.

I was already sitting on the examination table when the doctor came in. He asked me about school and squash, a sport he said he also played. The fact that we had this in common was comforting.

It wasn't comforting, though, when he looked at my x-rays and said both curves in my spine had progressed significantly. They had been around 32 degree curves, but now were 42 and 45 degrees. When I heard this, it almost made me sick. I found it scary that my back had somehow gotten worse even with the alternative treatments. Not only that, but I hadn't seen any noticeable change in my appearance.

"At this point, I recommend an operation." The doctor's words snapped me back to the present. "If you want to, however, you can get a second opinion."

I was terrified and started to cry. I felt like a pathetic mess sitting there on the examination table crying, but I couldn't help it. Ever since I was first diagnosed with scoliosis, I never really thought I'd have to have an operation. Dr. Drummond and my parents tried their best to comfort me. Mom held my hand and we all started to ask questions. Dr. Drummond even called me "sweetie" and put his arm around me. The reality of the situation really hit home when I heard my parents ask, "When should we schedule the operation?" And, "How is the surgery performed?"

Dr. Drummond said the surgery could happen whenever I wanted, although most people preferred to get it done over the summer. He explained that during the surgery, he would take two rods and use them to straighten my spine by cranking them, along with my vertebrae, into a straight line. He would then take bone from my hip and put it in my spine to help it heal. The bone, he said, would eventually "fuse" to my spine. At that point, the rods would be unnecessary. He said in rare cases, people could feel the rods when they sat in a chair and sometimes opted to have them removed. But that would mean another operation. So, in my mind, I ruled that out. It was really beginning to sink in just how serious an operation it would be.

Mom, Dad, and I walked outside where Dad hugged us goodbye and went to work. On the way home in Mom's car, she handed me her cell phone and suggested I call Grammy and Aunt Joanne. I remembered how much I had needed to talk to them when I had first been diagnosed. I was thankful that I had mom here to use her strategizing skills to help me get through this.

I called Grammy first. "Oh, honey," she said, "it's so nice to hear your voice." I could just picture her beaming because I was calling her. I told her why I was calling, feeling a little guilty that it wasn't just so she "could hear my voice." She was completely supportive. "It's okay. Don't worry more than you have to. We all have hard times." We talked for a while about family stuff, and I laughed when she told me a story about my three-year-old cousin's obsession with spoons. At the end, she told me she loved me and asked us if we would drive up to Massachusetts that weekend for a visit.

After I hung up, Mom "convinced" me that I should blow off school and go shopping with her and have lunch. Like she had to twist my arm!

We went into a few stores where I tried on tons of clothes, finally deciding on a pink boatneck top and a jean miniskirt. Then we went to a nearby restaurant, where I got a huge sandwich, french fries, and a big piece of cake for dessert. Nothing like food and a new outfit to make me feel better.

¤

That weekend, we drove to Grammy's house in Massachusetts. I was excited because I hadn't seen her in a long time,
and whenever I came to her house she liked to make delicious
banana bread. We stopped to buy her flowers because we
knew she was feeling badly about my operation. We decided
on yellow tulips, which I held in my lap for the rest of the five-
hour drive to her house.

When we arrived, she gave us both big hugs and kisses.
She told me I looked beautiful and said I had grown a lot. I
couldn't help thinking that I would have grown a lot more if
my spine hadn't decided to curve all over the place. Grammy
looked closely at my mother and said, "Well, you look stressed,
as usual." She winked at me and then smiled. She said she
was sorry about my news and that when she'd experienced the
same thing when she was young, she'd gotten through it fine.
"It seems scary, but you can do anything." And then, as if we
hadn't already hugged and kissed hello, she hugged me again.
I could tell she really meant what she said.

"Speaking of your recent news," she said, "you must really
be tense." She leaned close to me and whispered, "Maybe
even as tense as your mother." She smiled at us both. "So
to help you relax, I baked some banana bread. I'll go get
it. Come into the living room and sit down." She walked
down the hall to the kitchen while we went to sit in the
living room. In the sun-filled room were two chairs and
a sofa positioned around an old wooden table. The room
was decorated in various shades of blue and red and was
connected by a long hallway lined with artwork and family
photos. The rest of the house had three bedrooms, one for

my grandparents and two for guests, a kitchen, dining room, four bathrooms, all of it on two floors.

"Here you go," she said placing the steaming bread on the table along with some paper plates. Both my mom and I took a slice.

"Did I tell you I've been working on my photography?" she asked.

I somehow knew we were going to start off the conversation with small talk. My grandmother never rushes headlong into sensitive subjects. She brought out some photos and we passed them around. She loves taking pictures and is very skilled with her digital camera. She's entered her photographs in contests and has won a few prizes. As we were looking at a particularly beautiful picture of a bird and its reflection, I suddenly remembered the tulips. I excused myself and ran back to the car and got the flowers. When I handed them to her, she gushed about how beautiful they were and immediately put them in water.

She began telling us about her plans to take a summer trip with my grandfather. "We've been married forty-five years," she said. "I think we deserve a nice anniversary celebration, don't you? After raising your mother we need our vacations," she joked and we all laughed. "We're thinking Aruba," she continued.

The conversation then turned to more family talk, about my Aunt Joanne, Robert, and Dad, and how they were all doing. I asked how Grandfather was doing, and she told us that he was great, still playing tennis weekly at almost seventy years old. At just that moment, Grandfather walked in. As always, he was wearing a suit. He looked like he was in good shape, which I guessed was from the tennis. I thought about telling him that Aruba was too hot for formal dress, but I just couldn't envision him in colorful shirts and shorts. My grandfather is retired now, but he used to be the head of a big company. He is tall and thin, with gray hair that he keeps brushed neatly to one side. He charms absolutely everyone he meets, and it's obvious that he and Grammy are extremely happy. They have more friends than anyone I know.

He was surprised to see us. "I missed you women," he said as he hugged and kissed us both. "You, too," he said, winking at my Grammy. "You all look great. Why don't you visit more often? You know, I just came from a board meeting. Four hours long and really horrible if you ask me. They are all a bunch of stubborn old men. We never get anything done." Everyone looked as though they were waiting for me to tell him about my back.

"Grandfather, I have some news. You know my back? My scoliosis? Well, I have to have a little operation done." I surprised myself by adding the word "little." It was weird. I felt a need to console him, instead of the other way around.

"Oh, Elizabeth," he said. He looked sad. "I'm so … so sorry. That's terrible." I think he realized this might be making me feel worse, because he abruptly changed his tone. "You will do great, and guess what? Before you know it, it will be over and you'll never have to worry about your back again." Grandfather must have realized that I had come to talk to Grammy about her experience, because he told us he was going to take a nap. He repeated his encouraging words about my operation. Then he took a slice of banana bread, and said goodbye.

My grandmother clearly felt it was time to begin her story because she straightened up, patted her dyed blonde hair, and smoothed her navy pants. She was truly graceful in everything she did. She smiled and leaned forward. I was all ears.

"I remember the day that I was in my mother's bedroom, trying on a new outfit," she began. "I was standing in front of the full-length mirror and just as I was about to put on the new dress, I looked in the mirror. I could see reflected in it a bewildered and concerned look on my mother's face. She quickly regained her composure and said to me, 'Frances, stand up straight.'

"I was standing up straight. Or, shall we say, as straight as I could. What my mother saw at that moment was that my right hip was jutting out and my shoulders were uneven. My whole body was asymmetrical.

"Right away, my mother made a call to our family pediatrician to discuss her suspicions and set up an appointment to visit his office. Once there, he examined me, made me lean over, ran his hands down my spine, had me stand up as straight as I could, then confirmed my mother's fears. From this moment on, the word 'scoliosis' became a part of the vocabulary of my family.

"I was referred to a specialist, Dr. William Green, a world-renowned orthopedic surgeon at Children's Hospital Boston. I found him to be a very warm and kind man who did everything to make me and my parents comfortable. After examining me, he said that surgery was a possibility. However, he wanted me to try other preventive measures first, in hopes that an operation wouldn't be necessary. The first thing I had to do was to be fitted for a Milwaukee brace."

"Grammy?" I interjected. "At one point, the doctor had said I might have to wear a Milwaukee brace, too. Is it as awful as it sounds?"

"Oh, it's pretty bad, I guess. I won't try and sugarcoat it

for you. But if it helps you, then it's definitely worth it. In my case, I wasn't like you at all. I know you'll find it hard to believe, but I was rather shy. I was afraid that wearing the brace would turn me into some kind of spectacle. I felt people would always be staring at me.

"In thinking back on what it was like to wear a brace, one memory stands out. From the time I was seven years old, I went to overnight summer camp. The summer after I was diagnosed with scoliosis, the doctor said I could go to camp as long as I wore my brace and did my exercises. So I went, but when it was time to go swimming I would wait until everyone left the bunk and then I'd dash into the bathroom, take off my brace, put it in my duffle bag, and then run to swimming lessons. I would do the same thing after I came back. A lot of energy went into trying to hide that brace from my bunk-mates. But, of course looking back on it, I can't imagine they didn't know I was wearing it.

"But after all the months of wearing the brace, I still had to have surgery. There was great apprehension for all of us in the family as the time of my operation neared. First of all, it was not an operation that many other people experienced. We didn't have other families to talk to about it. In fact, we had never heard of anyone having this particular operation. Much like you, I had two curves in my spine. The doctors decided they were going to deal with the lower one first.

"First, I want you to know they've made tremendous strides in how they treat scoliosis. You'll no doubt have a far easier time of it than I did. The first thing they did after I was admitted to the hospital was to put me into a body cast of solid plaster. I was hung from a pulley to make me as straight as possible while a doctor wrapped me in the plaster. One of the differences with this cast was that it had a turnbuckle on the side so that as much correction as possible could be achieved. The plan was for me to be cranked a little bit every day. The more it was turned, the more the curve would be straightened, so they turned it as far as my bone structure would allow. I was confined in a cast and lost almost all mobility. It would turn out that my bed would now be my world for the next eleven months.

"After two months in the cast, it was sawed off, since it was time to perform the surgery. After the operation, I'd be placed in another cast until I healed. The spinal fusion would be stabilized with a graft from my left leg below the knee. The chips of bone were taken from the tibia in my left leg and wired to the lumbar spine to solidify the bone growth where they wanted correction. The hope was that once the bone healed, the back would be strong, resilient, and pain-free. They had to make a big slice in the middle of my back to scarify the bone so it would accept the bone grafts. The operation took a very long time and they had to give me enough ether to keep me under for several hours. You see, ether was the only anesthesia used in those days.

"After three months in the hospital, it was finally time for me to go home where I would continue my convalescence. There was a fun side to it, though. My house became the social center for all of my friends and even some kids that I was not friendly with. Every afternoon, groups of kids would come to the house and visit, talk, dance, eat, socialize, and just have a good time. It was *the* social meeting place for all of the girls and boys. My mother welcomed everyone. And so did I!

"I can still remember the day that I was first allowed to sit up and dangle my feet for a few minutes. A rush came over me. I was dizzy and felt like my head was going to explode. By this time, part of the post-surgery cast had been removed and I just had one that went from my neck to the top of my buttocks. I had someone support me on both sides, for there was no way that I could have stood up on my own since my legs were limp and wobbly. My feet were like jelly. So I had physiotherapy a few days a week, and slowly but surely was able to take a few steps and then a few more until I was pretty independent.

"When I left school to be operated on, I was in middle school and by the time I returned, I was in a high school. But the scoliosis wasn't done with me yet. I was being checked every few months and it soon became obvious my upper curve was getting worse. It was finally decided that in order to stop the progression, I needed another operation. The good news this time was that it could be done over the summer and I wouldn't have to miss any school. I could return to school in the fall, but I'd have to wear a removable body cast, which I did.

"When the healing process was all over, my posture was perfect. And eventually, there was no pain. I look back now and am proud of myself and what I accomplished.

"Well," sighed Grammy, "that's my story. But thankfully, Elizabeth, things won't be as difficult for you as they were for me. As I said, medicine has made such wonderful progress in this field. Thank God for that." She gazed directly into my eyes. I almost felt like she could see into them, into me. I was filled with such respect for her. She had faced such a terrible ordeal with such bravery. She was not even angry or bitter. I thought about how angry I'd become when I was diagnosed with scoliosis. And, at that time, I didn't even know I would need an operation. Grammy's story made me feel almost grateful for my situation. As we walked down the hall to sleep for the night my mother turned to me and said, "isn't she amazing?" I completely agreed.

When the weekend was over, I told Grammy I loved her and thanked her for telling her story. We gave each other hugs and kisses, and said goodbye. All the way home in the car, I didn't say a word. I was thinking. I wondered if I would have to face what Grammy had gone through. She had been so brave, so strong. Her story had been scary to hear, and I couldn't imagine what it would have been like for her to go through it. She had to have TWO operations. Yet I decided I would go through my surgery just as she had gone through hers. I did wonder though if I could be as brave as she had been. I also wondered how much it would change me and my outlook on life. As we pulled into our garage, I decided that as long as I had my family there to support me, I would be fine. I had to be.

CHAPTER EIGHT

My family and I trusted Dr. Drummond, but we all agreed that it was important to get a second opinion from another doctor. I'll admit there was a part of me that hoped a second doctor would tell me there was no need whatsoever for an operation. My dad decided to take on the project of finding me another doctor. I love my dad so much. He's always there for me. He is a cuddly bear—not the typical cuddly bear you'd imagine, although he does have brown short curly hair. He's thin and tall with a mustache and a small gap between his front teeth.

Dad's always looking out for everyone. He remembers the tissues you forgot to bring even though you have a cold. He answers the questions you have without your having to say them out loud. Everything about Dad and his thoughtfulness deeply affected my attitude towards the operation. He made me feel more protected and safe. It was Dad and his thoughtfulness that allowed me to go to summer camp. He's the one who realized I'd need to come in several months earlier than Dr. Drummond had recommended, because he knew that otherwise, if I needed an operation, I would have to miss my summer at Camp Walden. Besides being thoughtful and being my Dad, as a surgeon, he was the best person possible to find another doctor to ask about a second opinion for me.

He chose Dr. Betz at Shriners Hospital in Philadelphia. He was the President of the National Scoliosis Association! It doesn't get much better than that. Children flew in from all over the world to be operated on by him. Mom and Dad both went with me to the hospital to see Dr. Betz. We were directed to a huge room and over to some cubicles where a woman gave my parents a mountain of paperwork to fill out. As Mom and Dad worked on the forms, I looked up at a huge mural of handicapped children painted on the wall. There were red caps on the heads of the men in the picture and they were identical (only larger) to the cap that the monkey, Abu, wore in *Aladdin*. I later learned that these red, tasseled caps shaped like an upside-down pail were worn by the Shriners, the charitable society that funds the hospital. Their funds make healthcare at the hospital free for everyone.

When the paperwork was finished, we went up to the desk and the woman behind it began asking us a bunch of very detailed questions. I was beginning to get annoyed that the registration process was taking so long. When we finally got in the elevator, a young girl in a wheelchair got in next to me. I glanced at her and then, before the elevator doors shut, I looked again at the mural filled with the people in the Abu caps. I decided I was really rather fortunate and certainly should not have become frustrated over something so trivial as a bunch of papers and questions. Instead, I began thinking what the Shriners are doing is a great thing.

We waited in an upstairs exam room. It was smaller than the one in Dr. Drummond's office, and I liked it because it had less of that stuffy hospital feel. I got changed and a nurse practitioner came in to examine me. I was surprised at how nice she was. She made my whole family feel really comfortable. She told us stories about her job and her life. It was all so interesting I didn't even mind the checkup. She put my x-rays on the light board so we could see them clearly.

"How much pain do you have?" she asked as she got out a protractor and began measuring the angles of the curves in my spine. "My pain is not too bad," I answered. It really wasn't. I mean, once in a while I got a little achy, but it usually went away quickly. All she said was "hmm." It's one of those incomprehensible things doctors and nurses do just when you really want to know what they're thinking.

She then led us up to Dr. Betz's office. I think Dr. Betz had agreed to see me right away as a favor to my dad. The doctor shook my mom's and dad's hands and chatted with all of us. He was very nice and my concerns quickly melted away. So when he told me that he agreed with Dr. Drummond and thought I should have an operation, it wasn't too hard to take. Then he went more deeply into the subject of how the operation would be done. Afterwards he asked, "What do you want to know about it, Elizabeth?"

I didn't hesitate. "What will the scar look like?" I asked. This question had been plaguing me ever since I was told I might have to have surgery. Would it be small, like the one I had on my knee from biking? Or huge, like nothing I had ever seen? I was really curious about this, partly because I didn't want my back to look bad or gross, but also partly because I thought the size of the scar would give me a sense of how intense the operation would be. Well, I wanted him to be honest. Boy, was he honest. He brought up a picture on his computer of a woman's back with a pale red scar that went from her neck to her hip area.

"This is what your particular scar will probably look like," he said. "It will be very long, though no wider than a pencil." I tried to envision a row of pencils running up the center of my back. I didn't really know how I felt about the whole scar thing, except for the fact that it didn't make my stomach feel good. I wanted to be comfortable with my body and it would be a true bummer if the scar made me too embarrassed to wear bikinis or halter-tops.

My dad then asked about some technical stuff regarding the operation. To help answer his questions, Dr. Betz brought up another picture on his computer. It was an x-ray of someone who had just come out of surgery. The person's spine reminded me of the x-rays of my mouth I had seen at the dentist, x-rays of when I was wearing braces—yet this time, the hooks and wires were huge, the "teeth"—or, in this case, the vertebrae—were slightly curved and it was all sideways. The girl in the picture had a relatively straight spine with two vertical wires in the center of her back that were perfectly straight and latched onto the two slight curves that remained in the girl's spine. There were three sets of hooks, each set placed on either side of a vertebra, keeping the wires in place. There was something different though, metal pieces I hadn't seen before. Dr. Betz called these things "pedicle screws." He said these were put in between each vertebra on each side, a little farther out than the hooks, and they add strength to the wires and hooks on the person's back. If this weren't bad enough, he really frightened me with what he said next.

"I want you to know there is some small risk involved, Elizabeth. Because the spaces between your vertebrae are so small, installing the screws does carry with it the small chance of paralysis." He went on to explain, "If one screw is placed into your spine incorrectly, you could be paralyzed. But the chances are remote."

Part of me liked what he'd said about these screws, that they could speed up the recovery time in which my back would fuse and not need the wires. But when he said the word "paralysis," I trembled. I couldn't help but think of that mural I'd seen earlier of the children who were in wheelchairs because they were paralyzed.

Even though he was clearly an excellent doctor, I was relieved to get out of his office. Talking about the screws and possible paralysis had brought back all my fears. We decided to stop at the cafeteria to get something to eat, yet once there, I pretty much lost my appetite. The cafeteria was filled with sick children who were sitting at tables eating lunch with their parents. Some were in wheelchairs, and some others were using crutches. Seeing them was a reality check. At the moment, that world these children were in felt so far away, so far away from me and my life as I'd known it. Then it suddenly dawned on me that after my operation, an event less than four hours long, I would enter into that world.

My parents insisted I try to eat something even if I didn't feel well, and it seemed easier to go along with them rather than argue about it. I was so distracted, however, that I totally forgot what I was going to order when I was asked. All I wanted was to get the operation over with and get back to a normal life.

A few days later, I told Ali I was going to have an operation. We were having lunch and I just blurted it out. I needed to talk about it to a friend. While she reacted supportively, she wasn't exactly an expert at consoling. Ali looked shocked. "You're so brave," she said. "I could never do that. I would be so scared of death." This was not exactly what I wanted to hear, yet I understood where she was coming from.

I was also annoyed by other friends who didn't think about my feelings and asked me stupid questions simply because they were curious. One girl at school came up to me and said, "Are you going to die?" Another person exclaimed, "Wow, if I were you, I have no idea what I would do!" My favorite comment of all was when a family friend said, "Well, don't worry, I'll come see you when you can't move and are strapped to a board." What a jerk!

At least my parents were there for me. Everything around me seemed to be falling apart. I mean, all of the sudden I was going to be cut open with a chance of dying or being paralyzed. But my parents were so calm, I figured that I could relax, too. I decided to make myself believe that in the end, worrying would get me nowhere. (That, however, was definitely easier to think than do.) Mom told me I might as well get it fixed as soon as possible so I wouldn't have to worry about it anymore. She had a point. Another plus was getting my mom's full attention. She had stopped making as many calls on her cell phone.

¤

Two weekends before my operation, we went on a family trip to a beautiful inn in Connecticut for my grandfather's 70th birthday. In addition to my aunts, uncles, and cousins, Aunt Joanne and Grammy were there. It was comforting to see them, especially when I felt like I was up against the operation pretty much alone except for my immediate family. One of my aunts and I talked about the anesthesia. She said she'd had an operation in which she was put to sleep. My aunt said that it wasn't bad at all. In fact, she had no idea what was happening. That made me feel better.

Other family members asked me how I felt, yet tried to be sensitive about it. What was funny was that I was not really sure how I felt. All kinds of emotions were going through me as the operation drew close. I felt pulled in different directions. My emotions were flying everywhere. I was scared some days, and calm on others. I was happy some days that I could fix my back, and sad other days because I didn't want to have an operation. Some days I felt as if I were facing the operation alone, and on others, I felt as if my whole family and all my friends were there for me. The one thing I felt most of the time was that I just wanted to forget about it as much as possible. I kept thinking, why worry earlier than necessary about the operation?

At one point during this family gathering, I noticed that Robert wasn't enjoying himself as much as he normally did at these things. He's typically cracking jokes and making us all laugh. On this trip, however, he was quieter than usual. When we went to the movies, he didn't want to go along. He did smile sometimes, but the smile seemed fake. I began to worry about him. Every time I looked at him, he seemed to be staring off into space. I decided maybe he was acting detached because he was jealous of all the attention I was getting from everyone. It made me feel really guilty. I mean, I may "say" I hate him, but you can't hate your brother, especially when he is able to make you laugh really hard. So I finally decided to make it up to him. The next night, I told him we were going out alone for ice cream. We walked the dimly lit three blocks it took to get to the ice cream shop. I could tell he was puzzled as to why I was doing this.

"Okay, give it up," he joked, "you're taking me to a torture chamber."

"Hey, I'm just doing something nice for my brother. What's wrong with that? Seriously, I'm taking you for ice cream."

"All right," he said, smiling. Then, after a pause, "Fine, you're taking me to a torture chamber disguised as an ice cream parlor."

"Wow, you are *so* smart!" I said, laughing. He was acting normal again. I guess he just needed to get away from everyone.

When we got to Joe's Ice Cream, a large, friendly looking man we presumed was Joe sauntered out of the back room. Joe's shop was painted baby pink, and Robert and I joked quietly about how surprising it was that a big guy would choose such a feminine color.

The ice cream was lined up in a glass case with a dozen flavors. I got coffee and my brother got mint chocolate chip. I paid the $5.50, and we walked out. Even though I babysat at least once a month for our neighbors and got paid well for it, my money always seemed to disappear. There was always a good reason to spend it, and this time I decided getting Robert to talk was one of them.

"Thanks, Sis," he said, snarfing down his ice cream so that it almost fell off the cone.

"So talk to me. Are you having fun on the trip?"

"It's okay," he said slowly. "I don't know, Connecticut isn't really my kind of place."

I didn't know what he meant by that but I let it go. "Anything bothering you?"

He was quiet at first, then to my surprise, said, "Well, now that you ask, I'm a little worried about your back. I mean, it's freaky, you know? I don't know that much about it and I'm worried about you."

The way he said it was really cute and I wanted to hug him, yet I refrained partly because him yelling at me to let go would ruin our conversation and partly because I didn't want his ice cream all over my blue shirt. I suddenly realized that no one had really filled Robert in on everything.

"Hey, there's nothing to worry about. I'm getting an operation. Everyone gets them, that's why Dad has a job. And I have a great doctor, so it's fine. I'm getting rods in my back and when I come out, I'll be all straight. See? Nothing to worry about."

He smiled. "Thanks." I didn't know if he was referring to the ice cream or the explanation, but I figured maybe it was a combination of both. "You'll be fine," he said, and I sensed he was reassuring both of us. We walked in silence for a while and when we were almost home, he said, "Could I get scoliosis, too?"

I could tell this had been on his mind and I felt stupid I hadn't thought to tell him before. It was hereditary, what had I expected?

"Probably not, and hey, even if you do, it's much better for guys. Guys usually only get small curves and they rarely need operations." I knew the conversation was important and I felt we were closer because of it. I was definitely impressed by how well my brother was handling this. It made me happy to know he cared so much about me.

¤

I had a feeling getting ready for my operation would be difficult, and I was right. First, I was scheduled to meet with the anesthesiologist, a young woman with blonde hair who smiled a lot. When I first met her, all I knew was that I was having an operation. It hadn't occurred to me to think about what that really meant. I just accepted it, never thinking about what it might include—not that I even knew at that point. The anesthesiologist began by telling me that I would be put into a deep sleep and that there would be someone in the room watching my anesthesia and a neurophysiologist watching the electric activity of my spinal cord during surgery, telling the doctor where my back was especially sensitive, in other words more susceptible to paralysis. I realized that part of the reason I'd been so calm before was because I had no real idea of what an operation actually entailed. She, too, informed me there was some possibility I might be paralyzed as a result of the operation. I already knew this, of course, but it had always seemed to be such a distant possibility. When she told me, it finally sunk in and I knew it was a reality. I could go under the anesthesia and wake up afterwards unable to move ever again. Strangely, I remember thinking that if I did become paralyzed, I wouldn't suffer nearly as much as my family and friends.

To top it off, the woman who cuts my hair, Danielle, whom I'd told about my operation after I saw the anesthesiologist, said she was upset because her brother had just had back surgery at a local hospital and had lost the ability to move his legs. She said the doctors were trying to help him regain control of them. This story didn't make me feel much better.

Despite all this, there were other factors that were pushing me towards wanting the operation. Grammy called to tell me she'd run into an old friend who had been diagnosed years ago with scoliosis, but who had not sought treatment for it. The woman and her sister had let their scoliosis progress without treatment because at the time, not as much was known about scoliosis and their doctor told them they'd be safer if they did not have the operation. My grandmother told me that due to this decision, neither woman could stand up straight. They both had humps on their backs, suffered from severe back pain, and were forced to custom make their clothes and wear lifts in their shoes. I had never expected to want the operation. However, after hearing this, I definitely did.

A week or so after the appointment with the anesthesiologist, we went to see Dr. Drummond again. On the way there, I thought about how the rest of my life was in this man's hands. The idea creeped me out. I didn't like the fact that I had no control over my future. Although I trusted Dr. Drummond, it's hard to trust anyone that much. The first thing he told me really surprised me.

He said I should not expect my curve to be fully gone after the operation. Instead, he said, both of the curves would be around ten degrees.

Then he went on to say that we had some choices to make. He could do the operation from the front or the back. There was a downside to going in from the front though. Because one of my curves was so high up, he would have to get to it by doing a second incision through the front. We all decided to have him do the safest procedure possible, which was to only enter from the back. After the rods were put in, he'd put in crushed bone, so that eventually my spine would fuse and stay straight without the rods. We had to decide whether to take the bone from my hip or from my ribs. If he took the bone from my hip, the scar would be longer than it would be if it were taken from my ribs. If it were taken from my ribs, though, there was a chance of infection, increased pain, lung scarring, and perhaps difficulty breathing. Everything seemed to have a catch. I looked at my dad for guidance and he said, "I'd recommend choosing the lesser of two evils." And so after some thought my family and I opted to have him take the bone from the hip.

I was more than a little upset by this meeting. The decisions we made reminded me once again that although the technology was very good and had advanced a lot since Grammy's and Aunt Joanne's time, it was still not perfect and there was always a chance of complications. The fact that we were making a potentially wrong decision also scared me. I had always expected doctors to know every-thing, but now had learned because of the different analyses of my back by Dr. Ecker, Dr. Betz and Dr. Drummond, that nothing was certain.

Robert, who could tell I was nervous, started doing little things for me, like helping me carry my backpack and taking out the trash—alone and without having to be asked! When I was worried or upset, he would tell jokes and make me laugh. Once he came into the room dressed like a clown with a huge orange wig. Needless to say, this made me feel much better, as he sent me into uncontrollable laughter. One night, he got into the other twin bed in my room and asked me how I felt. It was so cute because he was only ten, and I knew that he was scared for me, too, and just was trying not to show it. He gave me hugs and was very supportive. I was lucky to have a brother who was actually brave enough to show me that he cared. He was brave in another way, too.

One thing I was really dreading was having to go to the Red Cross building and give blood, but I was told I had no choice. I was told I had to donate blood now in case I lost too much during the operation. Mom was also going to give blood so there would be enough. When the day finally arrived for us to donate blood, my mom, brother, and I walked into the building, only to see a dozen people sitting in chairs waiting to give blood, too. I already mentioned, I hate needles, so I was really nervous. It didn't help that there were other people in the room lying on tables and I could see the needles and I could see the tubes dark red with the blood passing through. My insides were turning inside out. Okay, I was totally freaking. Mom tried to distract me by telling me there was something great to look forward to after we gave blood—free food! It helped, though only a little. If before I'd been hyperventilating, now I was taking quick shallow breaths.

Our names were called and we were led to a small cubicle where a pleasant looking woman with a big smiling face was sitting in a chair. My heart raced as I sat down. I was thinking, *Oh, my God, how do I get out of this? There is no way that I am letting them stick a needle in me, much less keep it there for twenty minutes.* Just thinking about it made me sick. To top it off, the woman said my mom would have to go into another cubicle without me when she gave blood. Great! Goodbye, support system. This, however, was where Robert really came through for me. "Take a deep breath," he said, as the nurse took my blood pressure. "It's very high," commented the nurse. "Relax and don't be nervous." Easy for her to say!

Robert reached out and held my hand, but I still really wanted to get out of there. "We'll have to prick your finger," she said, showing me something that looked like an ear piercing machine, only in what seemed to be the color of the day—BLOOD RED. But instead of an earring back, there was nothing, because thankfully the needle didn't need to go all the way through.

The worst part was I had to do it myself because that was standard procedure. I thought it was cruel, if it was done to me I could at least count on a calm, reassuring nurse to do it. Instead, it was jittery old me who was going to hesitate forever. "Just count to three and do it," the nurse said. She had managed to gain a spot on my most hated list in under five minutes (an admirable record, if you ask me). I started to count, "One, two, three," but chickened out.

"You can do it," said Robert. I felt like the little engine that could, except I was the little engine that couldn't. "One, two, three," he practically shouted.

"OW!" It felt like an electric shock! The nurse took a thin plastic tube and collected some of the blood and then put a bandage on it. Wow, if that hurt that much, I was going to have a real hard time surviving the actual giving of blood. When she led me out of the cubicle, my heart started racing. "Oh-oh, this is it," I gasped panic-stricken. "I think I'm going to faint."

"No, you won't," said Robert. "You'll be awesome."

I got a hold of myself and laid down on a table just like the one in Dr. Drummond's office. I turned my head away from the machines and started shaking. It was like I was really cold and shivering, even though the room was hot. "Oh geesh, you're going white!" Robert said. "Just think about all the other people here doing exactly what you're about to do. Your strong, if they can do it, so can you." He paused, "You realize that your shaking so much the whole table is rocking back and forth."

"Then talk to me and get my mind off of it!" I said in a strained voice.

Just then, a young male nurse walked over. "Calm down, honey," he said. He was skinny with really white teeth. I got a mental flash of those ads for teeth-whitening strips. He gave me a hollow white tube and told me to squeeze it when I was asked to. I started to think about the needle and got scared again. He put some iodine on my arm and told me to breathe. "Oh, and stop shaking," he said with an even bigger smile. I just laid there silently. I didn't see how having a panic attack was funny. Then he showed me the needle and started tying something on it. When he was finished, the needle looked like a hornet with its wings flexed out. "Squeeze the tube," he said, while he tied a rubber glove around my upper arm. I wished he could hear my thoughts so he would know that I was mad at him for what he was about to do to me. "Just think of something else and you'll feel much better," he said as I glared at him.

"Talk to me, Robert," I said in a quivery voice. "Talk to me now!"

"Okay," Robert said, making a "that is gross" face at the needle. This was not helpful!

"Well …" Robert said hesitatingly as the needle went in, "… so how was your day?" Not helpful at all, I thought. I felt a surge of pain in my arm. "Talk about something else!" I shouted.

"So I went to school the other day and …"

"Hold my hand!"

"Ow," he said as I clutched his hand with a death grip. He smiled. "I hope you know there is no way that that needle hurts as much as my hand right now." This attempt to make me laugh did not work.

"Talk about something else…besides the needle!"

So he started telling me about people in school, and I answered forcefully with an occasional "wow" and "that's great." It was extremely helpful. A few times, I looked over at the needle and the bag but immediately had to look away, as I saw my blood being sucked through a small tube (I caught Robert doing this twice also and making a disgusted face). By the end of our conversation I felt like I was a member of their grade, based on the huge amount of random facts and gossip I had just learned from my brother.

Finally, the male nurse came back and announced I was almost done. But first, he said, they needed more blood and he told me to start squeezing the tube in my hand. I realized that I couldn't feel the needle anymore. Talking to my brother had made me forget about the needle! I'd gotten used to it. The forty-five people in his fifth grade class had gotten me through it. Actually, Robert had gotten me through it! He even got me to laugh when he told me he had challenged his grade's karate prodigy, an overachiever, to a fight and she flipped him on his back.

Then the nurse came over and told me to look away. When he pulled the needle out I sighed with relief. Robert did, too, and quickly left to go over to my mom's table where she was giving blood. I began to sit up, when the male nurse told me to stay lying down because getting up would make me dizzy.

I started to feel a bit better about the operation. I mean, if I could get through this horrible experience, then maybe the surgery wouldn't be so bad. My brother ran over when the nurse told me to hold his arm while he lifted me up. Wow, I definitely felt dizzy and a little weak. The nurse asked me if I was okay. Because I felt better, I said, "Yeah."

Robert helped me walk over to a long table where another man, who looked like he was my grandfather's age, was sitting. A woman handed me a basket of the free food my mother had told me about. I took a bag of chips and an apple juice and sat down next to the man and started eating. Food, glorious food. I felt like I hadn't eaten in forever. Robert sat down, too, and started telling me how impossible I was, how he was talking to me even as I kept on asking him to talk to me. I smiled, thanked him, and told him that I wouldn't have gotten through it without him. I meant it, too. I gave him a hug which he reluctantly accepted. He is, after all, a ten-year-old boy.

We had to wait there for about ten minutes after I had finished because my mom had started giving blood after me. The elderly man asked me why I was giving blood and I told him that I was having a scoliosis operation. He suddenly looked very sad. "You're lucky," he said, "not everyone in the hospital who's getting an operation, or who needs blood, has enough in the first place to save it for later." I decided right then that when I'm old enough, I'll try to give blood again. Although I'll probably have to drag Robert along when I do.

CHAPTER NINE

In seven days, I was going to have my operation. Grammy and Aunt Joanne called to say they'd be with me, which was comforting. I knew it would be a big help to have them there. I called Ali and we decided to meet the night before I went to the hospital. The days passed by faster than I could have imagined, a big whirl of tests, friends, squash lessons, homework, and wonderful comfort food dinners that my mom made to make me feel better. The next thing I knew, it was the day before the operation.

Mom, Grammy, and I went to the hospital one last time before the surgery. As we sat in the waiting room, a man walked up to us. He was almost completely bald, short, plump, and wearing a white hospital robe. He gave my grandmother a "look" and I realized, suppressing a giggle, that he was trying to pick her up. "Hey, do you have diabetes?" he asked in a sexy low voice that was the total opposite of what he was saying and looked like.

"No," my grandmother replied politely. And then, because she loves to joke, she added, "I happen to have high cholesterol."

The man feigned surprise and said, "Look at you! High cholesterol is impossible for a woman with your figure." He winked when he heard a nurse coming.

"Harry, come on. Stop wandering off!" the nurse said scolding him. She really sounded angry.

"Goodbye, ladies. Another woman calls for my affection," he said, returning to the sexy voice that had greeted us before he sauntered off.

"What a pickup line," my grandmother said in a low voice, imitating our newfound friend. The three of us started laughing. The woman behind the desk gave us a strange look and then told us we needed to go up to the fifth floor so I could give a blood sample.

We decided to use the stairs instead of the elevator and got lost by coming out on the fourth floor instead of the fifth. As we walked up the stairs my grandmother told me a funny story about my mom when she was little. My mom had apparently liked her first crush so much that she had followed him home one day on her bike. We all cracked up when my grandmother told of how she had gotten a nervous phone call from the boy's parents. Finally on the fifth floor, we found a door divided into two halves, with the bottom closed and the top open. You could see inside, where there was a room with a setup similar to the one at the Red Cross. I saw one of the nurses talking to a little boy who had just gotten some blood drawn, and then take a cylinder of it and drop it down a chute. I shuddered. Here we go again. I really hate this!

The nurse opened the door and let us into the room and asked who we were. Next, we were led to a cubicle where another nurse sat down and asked how old I was. She tied a thick rubber tube around my arm and started getting the needle ready. I started to wonder how I had survived giving blood at the Red Cross. I looked up at my mom. She could see I was terrified, so she asked me where I wanted to go for dinner. We'd just come from having a big lunch, but it didn't matter, because without Robert around, anything else was a welcome distraction, especially food. I felt the needle go in and had a flash of pain. "The Flume," I blurted out. "I want to eat at the Flume." "What will you get?" Mom asked, even though she already knew the answer, because I always got the same thing. "Prime rib, a baked potato with extra sour cream and butter, and a tangy tomato salad," I answered through clenched teeth.

"You forgot your Sprite," said Mom. "And bread. Let's see what I'll have. Probably the fish of the day with vegetables and a bite of your tangy tomato salad. Oh, and of course a big baked potato smothered in butter, just to make sure I completely massacre my diet." All of that food sounded amazing, I was dying to jump out of the chair and go. "You're both crazy," Grammy said smiling.

"You're done, lovey," the nurse said, taking the needle out. "Have fun at dinner," she added with a smile as she dropped my cylinder down the chute. As it whooshed out of sight, I calmed down. Mom's distractions had worked. We left and went back downstairs as my grandmother reminded me how lucky I was when we saw a little girl in a wheelchair roll by.

¤

Another major problem I had was that it's really hard for me to swallow pills. To make matters worse, liquid medicines usually make me sick to my stomach. I realized I'd better quickly learn how to take pills. I was pretty confident I'd be able to do it, because the summer before at camp, I'd gone to the nurse who'd given me two pills, saying they didn't have the liquid form of the medicine I needed. I tried to tell her I couldn't swallow them, but she insisted I at least try. I put the pills on my tongue, took a gulp of water, and felt them go down my throat. Success! Even though I'd done it at camp, when I tried to do it with vitamin pills about a month later, I ended up spitting them into my hand.

I knew I'd have to swallow a lot of pills, so my mom searched the Internet for the easiest way to get them down. She found a site that recommended you start by swallowing a tic tac breath mint and then an M&M. The idea was to start with small candy and work your way up to bigger candy and, hopefully, pills. My mom handed me a tic tac and a glass of water. Robert tried it with me. He swallowed his immediately. When it was my turn, I had so much trouble, the tic tac completely dissolved before I could even get it down. We eventually gave up.

A few days, later I tried again. I don't know how it happened, but this time I just didn't think about it and before I knew it, the candy went down. At least I'd done it once. The big question was, would I be able to do it over and over again right after the operation?

Mom, Dad, and I started thinking about what I would need and want during my stay in the hospital. Mom tried to get me assigned to a private room after the operation, and Aunt Joanne asked me whether or not I would want movies. Grammy offered to lend me her mini-TV with a DVD player to put in my room once I was home. Everyone was helping.

I needed to be kept busy, so my family and I went shopping. Mom wanted to make parts of all of this fun, and thought that if I had things I like, they would distract me. Of course, as one might imagine, I didn't mind these family outings to the mall.

We bought several different pajamas. I also bought a velour sweat suit in the exercise section, even though in the hospital I knew I'd be far from active. (I'd been told that I probably wouldn't even be able to stand up for a while.) There was also this cute flowery nightgown I loved, but my dad vetoed it since, he explained, it wasn't a good idea for the fabric to touch my scar or back. We went to a music store and bought two of the best CDs , *Best of the Grammy's* and a new John Mayer CD. I got four books, and was so eager to read them that I finished them all before I even stepped inside the hospital. Lastly, my mom got me these great fuzzy slippers! The shopping definitely kept my mind off the operation, but you can only get so distracted.

My grandmother and aunt arrived the night before my operation and that was great because they both love to laugh. We had a big family dinner and the mood was easygoing and comforting.

¤

The next morning, my alarm went off at 4:30 A.M. I got up and just went through the motions of getting ready. I was avoiding the thought of possible complications and the reality of what I was about to go through. I did think, however, I was going to be the most stylish patient there as I placed my blue slippers carefully face down on top of my new velour sweat suit. I added a toothbrush and a hairbrush, and was done packing. We all walked outside as my dad's parents drove up the driveway, punctual as always. They had agreed to take Robert for an overnight. Everyone hugged Robert. Before he got in their car, Robert turned to me and said, "You'll be fine." That's when I reached out and hugged him tightly. To my surprise, he hugged me back, just as hard.

We all drove in Dad's car, and Grammy and Aunt Joanne cracked jokes the whole time trying to distract us. At the hospital, we went to the special section reserved for children who were having operations that day. When we got out of the car,

I almost forgot my bag because I was so preoccupied. There was no way now that I could deny that all of this was really going to happen.

As we sat in the preoperative waiting room, a young woman and her mother walked in with a baby who was also scheduled for an operation that day. To our horror, the nurse told the mother that they would have to postpone the operation because she had fed the baby milk that morning by mistake. The nurse said she was sorry, but there was no way the baby could be operated on. The mother started to cry, yet there was nothing she could do. It was so sad because the baby was helpless and the mistake was not her fault. That brought to mind the same mistake I'd made before my MRI when I'd eaten the mango. I realized how lucky I was that I hadn't done it today. Now I really wanted this over with.

Later, after I'd changed into a robe and been given my hospital ID bracelet, a nurse called my name. There was nothing to do except get up and follow her. I turned around once and surprisingly, let out a little chuckle as I saw my grandmother's flash on her camera go off. She was documenting the whole thing!

Mom, Dad, and I went into a large room filled with rows of hospital beds, all on wheels. The nurse directed me to a stretcher in the corner and told me to lie down. A doctor came in and started to explain some details so that when I woke up, after the operation, I wouldn't be quite so frightened. Although they gave me a sedative which quickly had me dozing off, I do remember her telling me about the monitor I would have that would show me my heart rate, about the morphine I would be on, and about the needles in my arms through which the morphine and other fluids would travel.

Thinking about it now, I'm lucky she told me this as I was going to sleep and not when I was alert. At this point, the sedative was really kicking in, and I didn't even have the energy to worry about the operation at that point. I just kept getting sleepier and sleepier as Dad held my hand.

Chapter Ten

Since I was zonked out by the anesthesia, I can't remember the operation. All I can recall is falling asleep in that large room and waking up in a small room, lying on my back. Later, my parents said that I was in intensive care right after the operation. I don't remember much about it, yet they can—vividly. They told me that during the operation, they were in another room with my grandmother, my aunt, and the families of other kids who were being operated on at the same time.

They said a nurse came into the room every hour or so to give them an update. They were relieved to learn that the operation was going well and quickly. Three hours later, the same nurse came in and told them, "Elizabeth is asking for..." she paused. "Her glasses." The other families in the waiting room laughed, thinking it was funny that I had asked for my glasses before asking for my parents.

Ten minutes later, Dr. Drummond came in with the x-rays and held them up against the window to show my dad. He was very proud of the results, and told my dad that I wanted to see him. At that point, my mom jumped up. She wasn't happy being third in line behind my glasses and my dad! This got another big chuckle in the waiting room.

Dad came in to see me, then came out and got my mom. Since I was still under the lingering effects of the anesthesia, I guess it's not to surprising that I don't remember this at all. I was in a room with about twelve other people who had just gotten out of surgery, too.

My parents were so relieved that it was over and had gone smoothly, although my mom was horrified because my face was scabbed and swollen. Dad said this was because I was lying on my stomach and face for the entire operation. Later, I was a little upset because my mom lied and told me I was doing fine right after the operation. In truth, as I found out later, my heart rate had gotten very high causing alarms to go off every couple of minutes. My parents, especially my mom, had been terrified.

After the operation while I was in intensive care and was still really out of it, apparently I blew my parents a loud, theatrical kiss and yelled out, "MWAH!" (HOW EMBARRASSING!) And then I fell back into a deep sleep.

Next thing I knew, I woke up in the room where I would be staying during my recovery at the hospital. I had a sheet over me and my bed was flat, so I couldn't see a lot besides the ceiling. For a second, I panicked and thought I was in the morgue, lying next to a bunch of other corpses. When I realized the sheet wasn't over my head, it hit me that I must be alive!

I was able to move my head just enough to see that Grammy and Aunt Joanne were in the room with me. I was so out of it, instead of feeling excitement or sadness, I felt nothing. They kissed me and asked me how I felt. As they talked to me, I stared absentmindedly at their blurry faces (I didn't have my glasses on and my contact lenses were out of the question). We only talked for a minute but that took a lot of concentration and made me want to fall asleep. I don't remember them leaving before I fell asleep again.

Later, I clicked the call button and a smiling nurse came in and asked me how I felt. She seemed so nice, and I was really happy to see her, although that was probably partly from my morphine-induced mood swings. She said her name was Carla and told me if there was anything I needed, I should just push the call button. Carla also showed me another button on the remote control-like pad, which I could hardly see without my glasses. This button, she said, would give me more morphine when the pain got to be too much to endure. "You can push it as many times as you want," she explained. "It's designed not to let you overdose."

For some reason, it was hard to talk. Maybe I was just too exhausted from what I'd been through. I asked her for my glasses and she said sure. When she brought them and I put them on, my eyes slowly scanned the room, but I was careful not to move my head or neck. The room was mostly white, with a pink-and-green checkered pattern on the curtain that divided the space.

Carla told me if I got uncomfortable, I should just call her and tell her to come and roll me over. "Would you like a pillow?" she asked.

"No, thank you," I mumbled. I looked around the room again as she left. There were tons of balloons, and the room was filled with gifts I guessed were for me. The area was quite small. There was a cabinet on the wall in front of me, next to a plain wooden door I figured was the bathroom door. On my left, I could see an "attractive" green chair that had the foam stuffing coming out of the bottom. And on my right, there was another less comfortable-looking wooden chair and a metal IV pole. I looked at the pole and the bags and monitors attached to it, suddenly remembering that it had a purpose. My eyes grew wide when I realized I had needles poking out of both of my arms. It was gross looking, and I became a little sick as I realized that unlike the twenty minutes at the Red Cross, these needles weren't coming out for a long time. I later found out that I had a Foley catheter inserted to drain my pee, and that they wouldn't take it out until I'd learned to go to the bathroom again.

I was uncomfortable in a stiff, constricted way. It's hard to describe. It was as if I couldn't move as well as I used to because I was tired. I didn't have a lot of pain; though of course this was because I was on a morphine drip and still had some anesthesia in my body. Part of me wanted to see my family, but another part felt it was just nice to relax and not talk so much. Before she left, Carla told me to try and sleep.

Before I fell asleep though, it hit me. The operation had worked! I got this huge adrenaline rush and a great feeling of self-confidence and excitement. I wanted to do a victory dance, but the fact that I couldn't move was a bit of a problem. The excitement suddenly went away when I realized the operation was over but that the recovery part of it hadn't really crossed my mind.

Even though I hadn't eaten for about twenty hours, I wasn't hungry at all. My stomach felt queasy, but not like I was going to throw up. I slept on and off the rest of the day. After I was on my back too long, I started to get sore. I pushed the call button and the nurse came in and turned me on my side. I had to have her do that a lot. Sometimes, my dad did it for me and he was great at it. To be totally honest though, I wasn't always aware of who was rolling me over.

Carla was the first nurse I had and she was calm, professional, and reassuring. She had a way of making me feel confident about what I had to do. Carla's hair was platinum blonde, a perfect match to complement her long, silver and purple fake nails. But other than her focus on her nails and hair, nothing else got much attention. She wore no makeup, her hair hung in a low casual ponytail, and she wore loose baggy nurse's clothes. I admired her sense of self. She had a confident way about her that told the world she was paying attention to what she cared about, and if they didn't like it, too bad. She would roll me over every two hours with what she called a log roll, the standard roll where I would be stiff as a board except for a slight bend in my knees as she pushed my whole body over in one fluid motion. She would also come in from time to time to ask me how my pain was. When my mind was defogged enough for me to pay attention, I could really tell she took her job seriously and that she knew what she was doing.

Dad slept in the room with me the first night. We all knew this was going to be the hardest night for me, so his being a doctor would be a big help. I felt badly because I could sense he wanted to bond, but I just kept falling asleep and was too uncomfortable to talk. He had to keep rolling me over every two hours, so I wouldn't be in too much pain as my muscles got tired of holding my body in a particular position. He'd put his hands under one side of my back and legs and gently push me over. The next thing he did made him the best at it. He'd take blankets, roll them up, and wedge them behind my back. He made the blankets stiff so I could really lean on them, and this made a huge difference.

It is crazy to think that if I hurt this badly, how much more pain I would have been in without the morphine. This made me wonder how my grandmother, who didn't have morphine at all, had withstood the pain. It was almost impossible to think about.

Dad stayed up very late and just stood by my bed making sure I was okay. He eventually took a nap in the chair next to the bed, but had to get up when I started to feel uncomfortable, and needed to be rolled over, usually around 2:00 A.M. I would usually push the morphine button before I was turned over, because rolling over (or any movement for that matter) was a lot more painful than lying still. Not surprisingly, I couldn't sleep through the night. Dad said that whenever I was "awake," I was really half asleep. This was good, because I wanted to sleep constantly. When I was asleep both the pain and the strange woozy feeling went away.

When I woke up the next morning, my whole body ached. The anesthesia had completely worn off now. I was reluctant to move because every time I did, I got sharp pains in my back. My throat was really sore, too. Dad said that was because I'd had a tube down my throat for oxygen all during the operation. I knew I had a catheter for my pee, but I learned I also had another catheter in my lower back to drain the extra blood that had been left by my operation. A day earlier, this knowledge would have made me throw up. I guess I was learning that I could only be grossed out so much. When a nurse came in to take my blood, I wasn't looking forward to the needle, but was too exhausted and too used to things by now to even get upset.

Later in the day, Dr. Drummond stopped by my room. "You did very well," he said. My dad was there, and he and Dr. Drummond mostly talked to each other. That was fine with me. Sleeping in short spurts and having to roll over every few hours was a lot of work. I was tired. I was also in pain. I pushed the morphine button a few times, though to my dismay, it still hurt a lot. I then pushed the call button, but Carla didn't come. A new nurse, Gina, arrived instead. She had red hair she'd pulled back in a clip, framing her big eyes. My monumental accomplishment for the day was sitting up on the edge of the bed. When Gina came in she decided that this was the perfect time to try it out. I reluctantly agreed. First though, I pushed the button twice for morphine. It was important that my back not be twisted or bent, so I was rolled to my side. Next, Dad took my legs and Gina took my torso, and in one synchronized motion, they sat me up. I was like a toy soldier, holding myself perfectly still as I was moved around by others in swift movements. When I sat up I felt woozy and light-headed. I felt much dizzier than I had at the Red Cross. I never thought that sitting up would be so difficult. My feet were touching the ground and my butt was on the very edge of the bed. Mom was behind the bed, and my father and Gina were in front. They were there just in case I blacked out or started to feel pain.

It was weird. I was sort of zoned out and not interested in what was happening or in what anyone was saying. Finally, after about five minutes, it was time for me to lie down again. Dad took my legs again while Gina took my torso. I was supposed to be put down on my side and then rolled on to my back (the reverse of before). Gina, however, made a mistake by twisting me so that I went right onto my back. A huge bolt of pain shot through my back. It was the worst thing I'd ever felt in my life! I started crying. Gina was very upset, and apologized a lot. Even though I pushed the morphine right away, I was still in tons of pain and couldn't stop sobbing. They kept asking me if I was going to be okay. I told them the truth. I told them I'd felt something in my neck crack. "Oh, my God!" screamed Mom. She looked absolutely horrified.

Gina carefully felt my back and told me it was okay. It took a while, but eventually the pain subsided to a more tolerable level. It was a scary moment, but we all forgave Gina because, of course, she hadn't meant to hurt me.

During that first day following the surgery, the pain wasn't normally all that bad. Besides, I was out of it so much of the time that I wasn't miserable for extended periods. I'm sure that if I had been more aware of everything that was happening to me and how everything felt, I would have been really depressed.

¤

There was one major sign of how out of it I truly was: I had a TV in my room and not once did I ever turn it on. I also never listened to my CDs. I never felt like reading anything either. In the beginning, I didn't even think about Robert, or Ali, or my friends. The only thing I could think about was the pain.

Later on, I was given my daily medicine. I had to take codeine, another pain medication. It was a small, flat pill and I got it down somehow. I also was given a liquid laxative. This was because lying flat and taking pain medication made me constipated. I just gulped the red syrup down but afterwards, as usual, I came very close to vomiting. It tasted bitter and had the consistency of molasses. I asked Gina if I could have laxative pills instead of the liquid the next time, and she said I could. She warned me, however, that they were fairly large. I knew that no matter how large the pills were, I needed to swallow them so I would never have to drink the liquid laxative again. Practicing ahead of time with the tic tacs ended up being a huge help.

I was getting through each minute and hour, waiting for the second day to be over. The sleeping made it go faster, but the fact that I had to be rolled over every two hours was pretty horrible. My grandmother and aunt arrived in the afternoon. I barely noticed them and I felt badly that everyone went to all that trouble to be there with me and all I did in return was sleep. I tried to talk to them for a few seconds, but it was no use. I shut my eyes and dozed off.

Still, I really appreciated the fact that my family made sure that I was never alone. This was great for me in case of an emergency or something, but I know it was terribly inconvenient for all of them. They would come back and tell me a joke about the restaurant or cafeteria they ate in, but I wasn't really in the mood to laugh, so I just usually stared at them.

Sometimes, when I couldn't go to sleep, they'd talk to me and I'd just mumble "uh- huh" to the person. It was like I was having an out-of-body experience. When people would talk to me I would be half-listening, half-lying there feeling achy and queasy. It's hard to explain, but it was as if they were talking to my body while I was somewhere else in the room watching them all silently.

On the second night, my mom stayed with me. She took the second night because she wanted to leave the next two easier nights for Grammy and Aunt Joanne. I hadn't noticed it the night before when dad was there, but the beat-up green thing I'd thought was a chair was actually a bed. It was lower than my bed and it looked really uncomfortable. As Mom made it up with some sheets, she asked me how I was doing. She'd been so helpful through my whole experience. She'd tried so hard to make sure I wasn't nervous or scared about the operation, to the point that she helped plan distractions like the family trip for my grandfather and shopping outings. All the while, I knew she was hiding her own nervousness while trying to make me feel more calm and secure.

Even though over the years we hadn't spent as much time together as maybe I would have liked, my mom is one of my best friends. I tell her absolutely everything. Besides, she loves to eat and shop just like I do! More importantly though, when I need advice I always turn to her and believe me, her advice is always great. I always resented her job because she wasn't always there for me. The operation, however, seemed to be changing things.

I love it that Mom and I share so much in common. We often have long talks in which we analyze our lives. Lying there in the hospital bed, I wanted to tell her everything, about how miserable I was feeling. However, I was just too tired, and she seemed to understand. Amazing as she is, she's not a doctor like my dad is, so every two hours we had to call Carla to come in and turn me. One time during the night when Carla was busy, a large, strong man who looked like a professional wrestler walked in and asked me what the problem was. My mom told him I needed to be rolled over. He grunted something and then jerked me up and forcefully pushed two towels against my back. It hurt so badly, but I managed to hold my tears back until he left. Then, man, did I let loose. Mom put her arms around me comforted me, and I pushed the morphine button for a dose. I was so upset about the excruciating pain, I just wanted to get out of the hospital. I guess my emotional outburst scared Mom, because she asked me if I wanted her to call my dad to come stay with me instead of her. I told her no and closed my eyes. The night went by very slowly, with me drifting in and out of sleep. I think Mom must have been doing the same. I didn't want to keep her up, but she wanted to do a good job, so she stayed up as long as she could.

The next morning, I went through the same routine. Just like the day before, I had goals set for me. I was supposed to sit up, then stand. After this, I would sit up in a chair for as long as possible. I couldn't imagine doing this. But even though I was exhausted and still in a lot of pain, I was excited to get out of bed. Through this short trip and almost every other second of my time at hospital, the morphine sent me into a haze. At the same time, my body was working so hard to get better that I had almost no energy left. I didn't even have any sense of morning or afternoon although I knew that it was nighttime whenever everyone left besides my sleepover buddy.

Gina came in, ready to help me achieve my goal for the day. Nervous, I pushed my morphine button, in case anything went wrong again. She rolled me onto my side, placed a chair about a foot from the bed, then sat me up like she had the day before. I felt mildly dizzy, so I stayed in that position for several long moments before I felt ready to move on. Gina stood in front of me and put her arms under mine, and then she hauled me up to a standing position. I felt a small wince of pain that I decided to ignore. With Gina's support, I managed to walk slowly over to the chair, then sit down in it. My mother marveled at the perfect posture I had because of my stiffness. "Your back is as straight as a rod!" she said, which made even me smile. My entire family likes to crack bad jokes. I sat there for a few seconds, feeling disoriented, like I had when I stood up after getting the MRI.

I gripped the armrests and leaned back in the chair and tried to stay seated as long as I could, but forty seconds was about all I could handle. Gina stood me up with the same hold she had used before and helped me shuffle back over to the bed. She let go after I carefully sat down then she rolled me down and over the correct way. I was upset that the simple act of getting up and sitting in a chair was so hard. Time was moving so slowly.

The most comfortable position in bed varied. If I stayed in one position for too long I got sore, so I was constantly being moved around. On my side, I liked strong back support from towels and blankets (a pillow against my back was too soft to be comfortable). I couldn't lie on my stomach, so I would shift from my right side to my back to my left side, and then onto my back again. Once on my back, a pillow was placed under my knees to relieve the stress on my lower back. I was relatively comfortable most of the time, but not even remotely close to the way I'd felt before the operation.

Surprisingly, I didn't think about the fact that I had escaped paralysis. I was miserable, and therefore focused only on the moment at hand. Past and future had no meaning to me. All I cared about was just getting through each hour. It didn't require a large amount of mental power, because all I was doing was sleeping a lot or just lying down with my eyes open, thinking about nothing.

That night, I was glad to see Carla was back on duty and would be there to roll me over. Aunt Joanne, who was staying with me, had brought a bunch of cryptograms in a book shaped like a toilet seat. I was feeling a little better than I had the previous two nights, although better does not accurately describe the painful state I was still in. We did a few of the cryptograms together and somehow I managed to enjoy myself. Carla came back in and asked me how I was feeling. "Better," I said. "Then let's go for a walk!" she replied.

I was shocked. My monumental accomplishment for tomorrow was supposed to be a walk. I would be ahead of schedule if I walked tonight. I was nervous, but said sure.

"You go, girl," encouraged Aunt Joanne. Carla helped me stand up slowly. This was really cool. For the first time since the operation, I got excited because Carla told me that I was the first patient with my surgery to walk so quickly. I was ready! Carla was experienced and I really trusted her. Plus, my Aunt Joanne was there to help me, too, if I needed her.

I felt mildly dizzy at first, but was not going to quit. I pushed the morphine button and the three of us started walking in small, slow steps across the room. "You're doing great," said Carla cheerily as we reached the door. Outside in the hallway, a wooden banister was attached to the wall. My hand hovered above it, just in case. I was sort of walking by now. Okay, actually it was more like a shuffle. Each step took a huge amount of concentration and the upper half of my body was completely still the whole time. My body was so used to walking easily without even thinking about it. It felt really strange having to expend huge amounts of energy just to take a few steps. I worked my way around the circular hall, Carla by my side, and Aunt Joanne pushing the IV pole down the hall behind me.

It was funny because up to that point, I'd thought of my hospital room as sort of like a separate little house. I'd never been outside the room, so it didn't cross my mind that I was next to a hall or near other rooms. I'd felt quite secluded in my cocoon of a hospital room. But walking around the hall was also a perfect example of how, when people learn something new, it can change their whole outlook on life. So far my recovery had been my family, my doctors, my nurses and me. Now, however, I realized I was recovering along with many other patients. I wasn't alone. I also quickly learned I was definitely not the worst off.

The more I became aware of my surroundings, the more surprised I was by how oblivious and out of it I'd been. It's hard to explain so that it makes sense, but for a couple of days, I'd forgotten I was in a hospital. I sort of thought, without really thinking, that when my family left they stepped outside of my room and into the parking lot.

We continued walking around the corridor at a speed just slightly faster than zero miles per hour. I felt like one of those old drivers everyone honks at because they're going so slowly. I was thinking about this, shuffling along, when I started looking into each room as I passed by. All the patients were kids like me. Most of them were younger, but all were clearly sick. One girl had visitors and they smiled with sympathy as they watched me and my IV pole pass by the doorway. In the next room, a guy was walking on crutches, practicing his moves.

After I had walked the complete circle around the floor, we returned to my room where I laid down and promptly fell asleep. Carla came in when I woke up and wanted to roll me over. Before I was rolled, I could tell I was sore from all that exercise, but I soon started to feel better. I turned to my aunt and managed to say, "I can't believe I just did that. I felt like a kid learning to walk again."

Aunt Joanne smiled, "it's so weird to watch you go through this and remember what it was like for me. I was in a very bad mood while I was in the hospital, yelling at my mom and the nurses. The whole thing just kind of temporarily depressed me. I think you are definitely taking it more in stride."

"Thanks, but I've done that too. I still feel really guilty about kicking my uncles and grandparents out when they came to visit the other day. They drove all the way here just to watch me freak out."

"Oh, I'm sure they understand. You just had all your muscles and bones moved around and I remember that pain…its hard to imagine if you've never experienced it, but I bet they have a pretty good idea."

"Its just that I never thought about the recovery. Only the operation crossed my mind."

"I was the same way. It's kind of like you only think about what it is like to have someone go into your body and be all opened up, and so the recovery isn't as noteworthy because you'll be sewn up again." It was amazing how accurately she described what I was thinking.

"The funny thing is that it should have been completely the other way around. I was knocked out for the operation and the recovery is just like this slow battle that I have to give all of myself to fight."

"And you are definitely doing an amazing job, hon. You're three days out, right? Very impressive." I wanted to keep impressing my aunt but all of the sudden, I started to feel tired. I shut my eyes and fell asleep, waking up every couple of hours.

My aunt read for a while, then went to bed. She woke up a few times when I was rolled and eventually she fell soundly asleep.

When I woke up the next morning, my parents, Grammy, and Aunt Joanne were all in the room. A technician, the same woman as the first time, came in to take my blood again, but this time when she stuck the needle in, I felt a searing pain. I winced and she apologized, saying she'd missed my vein. *Well*, I thought, *this is great!* She put the needle in again and got it right, much to my relief. I then took my laxative and codeine pills and slept for a while.

A short while later, Gina came in and told me that I should try eating. "You can start off with some Jell-O or apple juice," she said. This was not appealing because ever since the operation, I'd had been fighting an underlying feeling of nausea. Gina brought in some apple juice on a tray and I drank it very slowly over a period of about ten minutes. Then all of a sudden I yelled for a basin and threw up in it. Even though nothing much came up, it really hurt and made me teary. Gina said that for now I should stick to ice cubes, which my stomach could easily take. I was worried, because I was doing so well with everything else. I knew full well I couldn't leave the hospital if I wasn't able to eat.

About halfway through the day, the two places where the IVs were inserted into my arms started to get red. I tried to ignore it, but they were really starting to hurt. I pushed the call button and told the nurse about it. She went and got two other nurses to come in and look at my arms. They gasped, and that wasn't particularly comforting. They said the needles used for my IVs were twice the size of the ones that should have been used. Everyone makes mistakes, I know that. But I like to think of doctors, including my dad, as superhuman and incapable of making errors. The nurses removed the IVs. I'd been under anesthesia when the needles had been inserted. I realized now that I was going to be wide awake when they inserted the new one. This was definitely not ideal! "Close your eyes," said one of the nurses, and with a quick sharp pain, the IVs went in quickly. It was over just that fast, and I was extremely relieved. I thanked them profusely for helping me.

After a little nap, my mom told me I was going to get a special visitor. Moments later, Dad walked in with Robert.

He was wearing a T-shirt and gym shorts, and I guessed he'd just come from squash practice. I could tell he was a little startled by my appearance. "Hi," he said. His eyes darted around. "Nice crib."

I smiled because my hospital room was more like a jail cell than a "crib." I was really sleepy, but used all my energy to pretend to be well and happy. I knew Robert would worry otherwise. In fact, I carried on the longest conversation I'd had since my operation. I tried to think of something to interest him, but it was like all my social skills had vanished in exchange for the rods and hooks in my back. I closed my eyes for a second. I didn't mean to, but I fell fast asleep. I woke up later and realized Robert had left. I was really happy to have seen him, and I hope he knew that.

Later on, Mom told me that my dad's parents, Nana and Papa, were here, along with my other aunt, Leslie, and her husband and her daughter. They all came in and gave me hugs. All of a sudden, I started to feel claustrophobic. I just wanted to sleep, I was so exhausted. So many people in the room at once made me feel confused and dizzy. I couldn't take it. Even though I felt guilty about it, I cried and told my mom I wanted to be alone. I think she felt terrible about asking everyone to leave the room so soon after they'd arrived. I fell asleep right after they left.

Later on that day, I went through the same routine I had with Carla the night before, except this time it was during the day and Gina was helping me. She rolled me over and I sat up. I was happy when I realized I wasn't as dizzy as before. I slowly stood up, this time without the help of a nurse, and walked out of the room. I was surprised at how different the hall looked during the daytime. It was lit up and the doors to all of the rooms were open. I got sad as we walked by a boy who looked about a year younger than my brother and who was wearing a Flintstones birthday hat. There was a huge sign next to this little boy's room, and it said "Happy 17th Birthday, George." *Seventeen?* I thought. He was finger painting and he looked happy even though he was all alone. I was horrified to learn he had AIDS and was slowly dying. I thought about this boy for the rest of my walk. If I'd had more energy, I would have run back and talked to him. Gina and I circled the hall three times and when we got back, I was so exhausted I collapsed onto my bed, still thinking about that boy.

¤

That night, my grandmother stayed with me. I knew the makeshift guest bed was not going to be comfortable for her, so I was determined to be extra quiet so she could sleep as well as possible under the circumstances. In true Grammy fashion, she whipped out a camera and took some pictures of my back and what she referred to as my "Miss America hospital hair." We laughed when she said this and it was then I realized how much better I was feeling.

In the morning, the woman who took my blood arrived and I cringed, remembering vividly how she'd missed my vein the day before. To my relief, she was successful this time. I figured this would be one of the last times I'd see her, because I'd been told that I'd be leaving soon.

Gina walked in with her trademark smile, carrying my red laxative and codeine pills. I swallowed them easily. And when she offered me an ice cube, I took it gladly. My heart fell, however, when I saw the tray she had brought in with

Jell-O on it. "You have to eat something before you can leave the hospital," she said. Dad handed me a spoon, and Mom said, "Just eat it quickly." Aunt Joanne and Grammy cheered me on like this was some big game. My stomach muscles tightened and seemed to be warning me not to push my luck. Nevertheless, I took a small bite and swallowed. I was discouraged to see the minuscule dent I'd made in the Jell-O. I knew I'd never be able to eat it all. Even though the cup of Jell-O would have been a mere snack before the operation, I wasn't hungry now, and this cup of Jell-O seemed like eating a whole second meal. I took three more bites and as my stomach started to churn, I told my family I couldn't eat anymore. Instead of enjoying food, I dreaded it. *What was happening to me?* I'd always loved food! At that moment, however, I felt as though I'd never want to, much less be able to, eat again.

Then it was time to remove my Foley catheter. I felt really awkward. Just another normal day in my new, not-so-normal world. When Gina got ready to remove it, I made an uncomfortable face. She looked at me and laughed and promised it would be quick. It felt like an electric shock, but in a second it was out. She told me that because I could now walk, I would have to go to the bathroom to pee, and to call her when I wanted to, so she could help me get up and down. She also told me to try to poop, because at the moment I was constipated since I'd been in bed for such a long time. I felt like a child being told about going to the bathroom. I remembered the time my great aunt had asked her fully grown stockbroker son—in front of everyone at our big family Thanksgiving dinner—if he had to "make a wee-wee." At least he didn't have to have a catheter. I cringed thinking about how it must work on boys.

I woke up a little later and another nurse asked me if I wanted to nibble on a cracker. I wanted to leave the hospital so badly by now, I forced myself to try. To my surprise, it tasted really good and didn't make me too nauseous. Somehow, after nibbling for an hour, the cracker disappeared and I was given another one. I ate that cracker, too, focusing on the shiny balloons in the corner of my room to distract me.

CHAPTER ELEVEN

The goal for the next day was to walk up the stairs, because the hospital wouldn't send me home if I couldn't accomplish that. A cute, muscular 18-year-old guy with a goatee walked in and told me he was there to make sure I was physically ready to leave the hospital. We walked outside together and rounded the hall. I was getting the hang of this, although I felt like the Bride of Frankenstein, which was a bummer since my instructor was great looking. For the first time, I noticed there was a belt around my waist with a handle on it that allowed him to grab me in case I fell. The nurses had always been behind me before and I'd been concentrating so hard I hadn't noticed the belt before. I felt sort of weird. I wasn't two years old or anything and now here I was on a leash. As we walked down the hall, my grandmother took pictures and asked me to wave to her. My helper didn't have much of a problem with this, although he probably would have if I hadn't been so comfortable with walking.

"Do you want to try going up the stairs?" he asked, even though that was the goal for tomorrow, the day I was scheduled to leave. I felt pretty good, so I said sure. We went into a concrete stairwell where he told me to hold onto the railing and to take it one step at a time. As I tried to lift my leg onto the first step, I was surprised at how hard it was. I figured it was just because I was so weak after the operation. Instead of putting one foot on a step and then the other on the next one up, as I would normally have done, I put one foot on a step and then brought the other up so that I was standing with both feet on the same step. Each time I lifted my leg, it felt like I was lifting a bag of cement. The whole thing was making me slightly dizzy. It was funny because my mind was ready to walk up the stairs normally, but my body had to stop and relearn how to do it. I only walked up about five steps and then down. But by then, I was exhausted, so we walked back with my family trailing behind. When I was finally back in bed, the guy told me I had done great and was a full day ahead of schedule. My whole family grinned as though I'd won some championship trophy.

A little while later, a nurse came in and told me they were going to give me a transfusion of the blood I'd had taken at the Red Cross. She said the transfusion would give me more energy and stamina. The idea of more energy and stamina excited me because although I had enough energy to do my daily tasks, I was exhausted once I finished them. A bag of blood was put on my morphine stand and it went through one of my IVs. Before the operation, I would have been so much more afraid and grossed out by seeing the dark blood flowing into me. I thought of my trip to the Red Cross and how at that time I'd had no idea of what I was getting into. I never thought I could do something like this, and for the first time, felt a sense of pride for having made it.

The nurse told me now was a good time to get up and go to the bathroom. I wondered if I would even have to go once I got to the bathroom, because I'd only nibbled on crackers and sipped a little apple juice. I stood up and dragged my morphine pole, still with the blood bag on it, and walked into the bathroom. The nurse did the fainter's hold, her arms under mine. With her help, I slowly sat down on the toilet, and then she went outside and closed the door. She said she'd be right outside if I needed her. I'm not used to having someone sit me down on a toilet. It made it a public event, which was really awkward. I'd been warned that I'd be constipated out of my mind, even with the strong red laxative pills I had to take every morning. I sat there, but nothing happened, so I called the nurse back in and she stood me up. Suddenly, my jaw dropped and I couldn't move! She saw the look on my face and asked what was wrong. I was unable to lift my arms, so I couldn't point at my horrible reflection in the mirror. I had small scabs under my eye and in the center of my forehead. Worst of all, my hair was like a beehive. It was in a loose ponytail on top of my head, forming a bob of hair that looked like small animals could live in it. It was so frizzy that it reminded me of wild straw. I was mortified! I suddenly thought of all the people who'd come to visit me. I had thought I looked bad but not *this* bad, not like an actual monster. Until that moment, my appearance had been the least of my worries. I was humiliated!

"Could you help me with my hair?" I asked the nurse. "It looks horrendous."

"Honey, it looks fine," she said. "Don't worry though, I'll be happy to help you brush it out." We walked back into the bathroom and she took out a brush. She supported my arms as I tried to pull out my hair tie, but even with her help it killed to lift my arms. The tie was firmly stuck in the huge knot that was my hair. The nurse finally pulled it out, having to rip out a clump of hair still knotted on it. She took out a cylindrical hairbrush and started at the ends. My hair was not up anymore yet because it was such a knotty mess, it sort of stayed in the same upward position. She started at the ends and each yank hurt a lot. She asked me if I wanted her to go softer, but I told her I was fine—I was desperate to get my hair back to normal. It probably would have helped if I'd taken a shower and washed my hair, something I had not done in four days. She yanked and pulled and worked her way from the bottom to the top. Finally my hair was unknotted, yet it was far from the healthy bunch of shining hair I had hoped for. It was more like a frizzy, disgusting mess.

I got back into bed and drifted off to sleep and a little while later my mom came in and told me that Robert was here to see me again, and would stay with me while everyone else went to lunch. The first thing he said when he saw me was, "I see you've managed to tame the beast." I knew immediately he was referring to my hair.

"Why didn't you tell me it looked horrible?"

"I didn't want to make you more self-conscious than you already are. You look fine though." It would have helped if he hadn't smirked when he said that, however.

When Grammy, Aunt Joanne, mom and dad got back from lunch, Dr. Drummond stopped by, and asked me how I was doing. I told him I was doing pretty well. I sat up on the edge of my bed and showed him the scar. He was impressed at my recovery rate and told me that if I wanted, he'd let me go home today, a day early. When he said this all I could think was, finally! Yet then I hesitated. I didn't know what would be best. I was definitely scared that the car might go over a bump and jar my back. My mom really wanted me to go home because she thought I'd been stuck in the hospital long enough. I decided to follow her advice and leave. Dr. Drummond said that was fine, though I would need a quick x-ray first just to make sure everything was okay. A nurse I didn't recognize walked in, said hello, and told me she was going to take me for my x-ray. She left for a moment and returned with a wheelchair. I asked her why I couldn't walk and she told me it was too far away. As she lowered me into the chair, Robert asked if he could follow with my IV pole. The nurse said that would be fine. Since I knew I could walk, I was a little embarrassed to be in a wheelchair. Then Aunt Joanne cracked, "Check out those rims!" We all laughed, including the nurse, and then we were off. I was surprised by the sunlight, which I realized I'd not seen since before my operation. It was really bright and made me squint. We went into an elevator as Robert talked to me and the nurse. It was funny, watching him maneuver the pole around corners, talking nonstop and running after the nurse, who was pushing my wheelchair quickly.

The x-ray room reminded me of the rooms I usually went in for my check-ups with my doctor. The first x-ray was relatively easy. The x-ray technician told me to put my chest up against a board and to hold my breath. I heard a click and that was that. Then he told me that I would have to raise my arms so that they were straight out in front of me. I tried, but it hurt a lot, and I only could lift them halfway. I was really disappointed when I had to let my arms drop. The nurse asked Robert to hold my hands for support. "When I say *go*," she said to Robert, "lift her arms. Elizabeth, you clasp your hands at the same time." I heard "Go!" and Robert lifted my arms as I put my hands together. Even with Robert's support, it hurt severely. I felt like crying as wave after wave of pain ran up and down my sides. The nurse said "Done!" and I let my arms drop. I was so happy it was over and thanked Robert before I sat back down in the wheelchair. If I'd had the strength to, I probably would have hugged my brother, but I was too tired.

We went back to my room and I lay down. Since I would be leaving soon, my IVs were removed and my mom helped me into my velour sweatpants and a T-shirt. I hadn't even worn my sweats once, even though I had thought I would every single day in the hospital. The nurse told me the internal stitches I got would dissolve and that the tape on my scar would fall off on its own. I felt like a present being taped up. I just prayed I wouldn't rip open.

When we left the hospital, I was startled. I had totally forgotten how beautiful the world was. The sky that day was bright blue, and the sun felt warm on my face. I had been in a dark hospital room for so long that now it was amazing just to be breathing fresh air. I felt a burst of joy, which made me want to run around and play even though I could only roll back and forth in my wheelchair.

My dad and the nurse rolled me down to the parking lot where my Grammy's car was waiting. We got in and my dad drove home. He knew that it was extremely important not to go over bumps because that would be painful for me. Still, I was scared to death. Everyone tried to distract me by talking about anything, like how nice the scenery was. Each time he saw a bump coming, Dad would warn me so I could brace myself. When we reached our house, I felt like I was finally coming back from a long vacation. I was so happy to see my home. It seemed as though I'd been gone for months.

When we arrived at the house, I was frightened to move. My muscles were stiff, and I didn't want to turn my neck too much. Since our driveway was made of gravel, it wasn't as predictable as the hospital's paved parking lot. I took small baby steps so I wouldn't fall. When I got to the house and stepped through the doorway, I was astonished. Everything seemed so much shorter and lower down than it had been before. When I told my family that, they thought that was really cool. I had grown two inches when they straightened my spine! I have to admit that being taller is pretty great.

I walked very slowly up the stairs and my father helped me get into bed. I looked over and saw the TV with the DVD player that Grammy had loaned me. I was pumped to watch the three teen movies—*Pretty in Pink, Sixteen Candles,* and *The Breakfast Club*—from Aunt Joanne. I thought about watching one now, but I was too physically spent.

As I lay there, I began to wonder how my school friends were doing. I was a little jealous. They'd probably been having fun while I was going through all the pain and stuff at the hospital. Regardless, I was so glad to be home. My mother had been right—I needed to get out of the hospital. I was so cooped up there, especially those last few days. But I was extremely proud to be the first scoliosis patient to leave the hospital so soon after surgery.

The pain had brought me to tears on many occasions, but I'd taken it hour-by-hour and gotten through it. I was happy and I was proud. I looked around and told everyone how beautiful everything looked. "Sometimes you don't appreciate something until it's gone," said Dad. He was right.

Aunt Joanne came into my room to say goodbye and said she had to go back to New York. She'd been there for me throughout my entire hospital stay. I smiled thinking of the fun cryptograms we did in that ridiculous toilet-shaped book she'd brought. She was just about the only one who could make me laugh when I was in so much pain. I knew I'd miss her. Grammy, however, would be staying for one more week to take special care of me, and that made me happy.

The hospital stay was over but because I had no nurses at home, I was warned that the next section of my recovery would be difficult. My parents had to go back to work, so it would be just Grammy and me in a big, empty house. Although I was worried that my dad would not be there to roll me over properly, I knew Grammy had watched him carefully and would do the best she could. And since I was finally at the point where I could actually carry on a conversation, I was looking forward to bonding more with her.

The next morning, my parents came up to my bedroom and I reluctantly hugged them goodbye before they left for work. I watched them bend down over my bed to hug me. I cringed when I thought of the excruciating pain doing something as simple as that would cause me if I were to try it. I didn't want them to leave, even though I knew my grandmother would be there.

The pain was a constant reminder that, although I was out of the hospital, the surgery had been just five days ago and I had a long recuperative period ahead of me. I was supposed to take codeine pills in the morning for pain, though the nurse wanted me off them as soon as possible. When I heard this I began to wonder why. Dad explained that they could really be addicting. He said that if I didn't absolutely need to take them, I shouldn't. This made me realize how strong and intense my pain medication really was. The morphine I was on in the hospital must have been even stronger. Though I took one codeine pill that morning, I was determined to stop taking the pills as soon as possible. Getting back to normal and having a healthy body were more important to me than ever, and pain medication wasn't part of my plan.

When I left the hospital, I was given a very interesting sheet of paper. It told me when I would be able to do certain things. It said I'd be allowed to swim in a couple of weeks, yet my true passions, squash and tennis, would have to wait until six months later. It also said how many pounds I could lift and when. It was helpful, but as my recovery progressed some of the limits got really annoying.

CHAPTER TWELVE

That first week home, Grammy and I accomplished a lot. Each night, I would sleep in my own bed, being turned often but much less than when I was in the hospital. Since there was no nurse to come every two hours, I was turned every four to six hours. In the daytime, I would slowly shuffle down the stairs and log roll into my parents' bed. This was because they have the most comfortable bed in the house. I loved to go downstairs. Being upstairs in my room all the time was just too restricting.

From my parents' bed, I watched a lot of TV. Even though I loved TV, I started to get bored with it. I was thirteen years old, and you can only watch so many episodes of *Blues Clues* and *Dora the Explorer*! I would sleep on and off and when I had to turn on my other side, I learned to help my grandmother by either putting the pillow under my knees or behind my back. I gradually started becoming more self-sufficient and more like my old self.

In the hospital, I had felt withdrawn as I was expending all of my energy just to deal with the pain. Now though, I was able to have conversations with Grammy and do a few things with her. We did a lot of cryptograms together, something I'd developed a taste for in the hospital with my Aunt Joanne. Grammy and I still do them today and they've become one of our "things" we share. I definitely felt better and more alive than when I was in the hospital, but I still was exhausted and slept nearly 21 hours a day.

As the days went by, I felt better and better. Whenever I was awake and moving, my back actually felt perfectly straight. Still, I was terrified to move my head or neck too much because I was afraid it would hurt me. I began to worry that I'd never get back to normal, that instead I would always look awkward and extremely tense.

¤

Ali visited me shortly after I got home. She looked very pretty, dressed in a new tank top and shorts. I have to admit, she brought me the cutest stuff and I did like the huge two-foot tall "We Love Elizabeth" card she'd gotten everyone in my grade to sign. She also gave me socks, a teen quiz book and lotion.

We talked about school for a while and after she left, I couldn't get my mind off of going back to school myself. I decided I'd left at the perfect time because I didn't have to come back in the middle of the school year and face more awkward questions like I had before my operation. I knew some people didn't understand how serious the operation was and never would. My other school friends, however, friends who took the time to visit me, definitely did. I really appreciated their stopping by, because I must have looked tired, stiff, and clearly in pain. The fact I couldn't get out of bed easily must have shocked most of them. Even though I felt better than when at the hospital, I still got sharp pains and needed to take codeine more often than I wanted to.

It was also hard for me to get dressed, so I preferred wearing things that were easy to put on and take off, like the robes I'd worn in the hospital. It was funny when I remembered how much I'd once disliked them and now here I was loving them because I could tie them easily in the back. Grammy and I finally came up with a solution and took a bunch of my dad's large jean, long-sleeved, button-down shirts. They were soft and light blue, and came down to the middle of my thighs. They were easy and comfortable to wear. I'll admit they weren't the most stylish articles of clothing I'd ever worn, but I was looking for comfort, not to make a fashion statement.

I also had to get through an important milestone—taking a shower. Looking back, I can't believe I didn't shower or bathe for a week and a half. Just the thought of it was repulsive and totally embarrassing. I did have a valid excuse. I couldn't step over a bathtub rim because my dad was worried I would fall. Because most of the showers in our house are in tubs, I had to use the shower stall in our guest room. Grammy laid out a towel and told me to call if I needed her (I guess in case I fell down).

It was more than just not showering when I was in the hospital. I don't remember ever thinking about my hygiene while I was there. I mean, I didn't even—*yuck!*— brush my teeth, though this wasn't as bad because I really didn't eat anything. I must say the shower I took in the guest bathroom that day was the best shower I have ever taken in my entire life. I couldn't shave my legs though, because I couldn't bend down, and I had to be really careful when I shampooed my hair, moving my hands as slowly as possible. I also couldn't wash my legs, as you might expect, since I couldn't bend. So even though this was not the most effective shower, it was much needed. I then put on one of my dad's blue shirts, buttoned it up, and laid down on the bed. My back was starting to ache from all of the activity that I had just gone through, even though it was just a shower.

¤

Unlike some kids, I really care about my schoolwork. In the hospital, I was preoccupied with the pain and with getting through my ordeal. Now that I was home though, I couldn't ignore how far I had fallen behind. I'd missed a whole unit on Greece in English class (including a paper), a unit and test in Science on winds and pressure, not much in Spanish, and a lot in Civics class. Math was a different story. Math is my best subject and so instead of missing anything when I went back, I caught up with the class and was fine. I had known that I would miss some school and thought that I might enjoy my operation break. I'd also heard other girl's stories in which they said how nice it was to be off from school for so long. Truthfully though, I was too busy at home with other things to think about free time. It's weird, because I really had nothing scheduled, yet I always felt overwhelmed with the basic stuff I had to do. The littlest chores became major undertakings. Even having a snack took a lot of planning and figuring out, which took Grammy and me by surprise.

Before, when I'd first learned that I needed the surgery, I'd focused on the actual operation so much, I never really thought about the recovery time, so I was amazed when I realized this would be the hardest part. Even my mom told me she barely considered that there would be a recovery period. We thought that when they let you out of the hospital, you were all better. So I was really happy that Grammy was there to help. She's very understanding and a terrific listener. She said it was a lot of fun taking care of me. I'm not sure she was being honest because I could see it was hard work for her. It probably wasn't great for her that she had to relive her operation through me, so it is even more amazing that she was so supportive. Our already unbreakable bond grew even stronger in that one week, stronger than it had in all the vacations we had spent together combined.

It was interesting to watch my progress. Grammy was about the only other person besides me who really recognized every accomplishment I achieved. I needed to gain back the weight I'd lost from the operation, because I was only 88 pounds after I left the hospital (including the metal in my back!). And since I hadn't been able to keep down food while there, besides crackers and ice, it was important for me to start eating now that I was home. I started out with small things, like fruit and juice, and one day I tried a bite of a sandwich. I ate it slowly and carefully and was ecstatic when it stayed down.

I also had other goals to achieve. I had to get up and move around regularly during the day. Grammy and I would go down stairs and go into the kitchen with its big floor-to-ceiling windows and sit down. Each day, the walks got a little easier. Sometimes, I would sit in a chair for fifteen minutes or so. It was funny how things I'd taken for granted before the operation had now turned into almost impossible goals that I had to work hard to accomplish.

I remember once thinking during my recovery that this is how it must feel to have Alzheimer's. I know it's a strange way to look at it, and granted I wasn't losing my memory, but I could tell that my brain was in a haze. It was like it was out of my control. I hated the feeling. I was mentally and physically exhausted a lot of the time. Grammy said that it was the same for her after her operation. It did get better, she said, but it took almost a full year. I didn't know how to make myself feel energized and focused. All I wanted was the light feeling of happiness and the carefree, fun life

I had had before. I had smiled since having the operation, but I hadn't laughed hard. I love to laugh! Now all I could muster was a weak grin to make a relative or friend happy. I wanted my old self back.

I guess I was just really cautious about getting too excited about anything because I wanted as little pain as possible. It wasn't just that I was exhausted, my personality seemed to have shifted. Unlike before, I now felt more reserved. I think it's because I felt I had to focus all of my energy on me and on getting better, and I didn't want to share my feelings with anyone. I can't really say why. I think I was just so tired that I didn't want to waste the energy to express my feelings. As a result, I became very quiet and only spoke when necessary. A few times, I had that weird out-of-body experience again, the same as I'd experienced in the hospital when too many people were in my room. I started detaching myself from situations. One way of describing it is that I felt as though I was looking at a play rather than a real-life situation.

A few times after Robert came home from school, he sat by my bed and hung out with me. We would talk and watch movies. Listening to him talk about school was really difficult for me though, because by this time, I couldn't wait to get back. I'd been home ten days and was supposed to wait another whole week. Still, I decided I was ready to go back to school for a short visit. That way, it wouldn't be quite so awkward when I went to class. So the next day, my mom drove Robert and me to school and I walked in and started hugging all of my friends.

They were all amazing! They hugged me carefully so as not to hurt my back. It was great to see everyone and it was fun to see Ali. We hugged each other the second I entered the building. I thanked everyone around me for signing the card Ali had brought to me. One of my guy friends came up to me and said, "that's so cool that you did that" and I felt proud.

My parents told me I could only stay for one class each of the first couple of days. Dr. Drummond had not given me permission to go back to school yet, and my parents were concerned that I might fall and get hurt. I was worried that if I sat for too long without lying down, it would be painful. Still, I couldn't wait to start all my classes again.

The very next day, Mom drove me to school for my first class. She kept on asking if I was excited and I truthfully was. I was getting bored and I wanted my normal life back. I thought that going to school would help make this happen. I was more than a little self-conscious though, because I had to move so slowly and stiffly, and I knew I looked a lot different than before.

The first class was science, one of my favorite classes mainly because my teacher, Ms. Michel, makes science so interesting. When I walked into the classroom, everyone was reviewing for exams. I was really embarrassed because they all looked up and stared at me. I sat down and tried to pretend things were normal.

I remembered the doctor had mentioned that after the bone fused in my back, the rods wouldn't be necessary anymore. He told me that in some rare instances, a few of his patients didn't like the feeling of the rods in their back, especially if they were thin and that in these cases, they sometimes chose to have them surgically removed. As I sat there in that hard desk chair at school, I could feel the rod in my back pressing against the chair. I thought about what he said, but decided I would not let it bother me.

When Ms. Michel told everyone at the end of class to put their stools on the tables, she added, "That is, except for Elizabeth." I was mortified. I had expected that when I went back to school, everything would be the same, even though it would be awkward. Right away, I realized this was not the way it would be.

After this, I just got back into the groove of school. I was told that if I was ever sore or uncomfortable, I should go to the nurse's office and lie down. I did this a few times. But when I did, it was for only fifteen minutes.

At the end of the school year, I studied my brains out preparing for the exams and aced the tests. A few days after school had ended for the summer, I went to the neighborhood pool to hang around with Ali. I could tell she was scared about my back because I'd told her I wasn't allowed to dive or jump in the water because of the impact it could have. Instead, I had to awkwardly slide into it. Even with all the precautions I had to take, Ali and I still ended up having a blast. I was not going to let my operation get in the way of a good time. I went to the pool another time with Robert and after a fight, he decided to jump off the diving board just to rub it in my face that I couldn't dive or jump. That's when I knew people were starting to see me as almost normal again.

I went swimming in the lake several times when I was at my eight-week sleepover camp in Maine that summer. I had an amazing time there, although I did have to be careful and put extra sunscreen on my scar. I also couldn't water-ski or horseback ride. But I was with my amazing camp friends and the summer was just as fun, if not more so than the ones in the past.

I recently returned as a freshman in high school and despite having to start the year off with a rolling backpack, I'm having a year that is really exciting and basically not at all affected by my back.

Just when I had begun to let my condition and experience slide to the back of my mind, my mother told me I had the six-month postoperative appointment with Dr. Drummond. The appointment was to make sure everything was okay. I started to worry, thinking that if there were a problem, I might have to repeat the entire ordeal.

Seeing Dr. Drummond brought back many memories. The whole experience was emotionally overwhelming. He started pushing on my back muscles. I was very proud—and not just a little relieved—when he told me how impressively strong and healthy they were. I then went and got an x-ray. Each curve had worsened two degrees, but apparently it's normal for scoliosis to get a little bit worse even after the operation. The really good news is that I'm almost done growing, so it shouldn't progress enough to pose any type of threat. Before I left, Dr. Drummond told me I was just fine.

¤

I'm proud of my operation. I know that sounds funny, but I think it makes me feel unique. And it's created a wonderful bond between my Aunt Joanne and me, Grammy and me, and yes even my brother Robert and me. As for Mom and me, it made us realize our relationship was more important than any job. It also deepened my bond with my Dad and Ali.

When I was diagnosed with scoliosis in seventh grade, I suddenly became different from my classmates. At first, that was hard to take. After having my spine straightened through surgery, I realize now that my personality may have changed even more than my back did.

I'm a much more determined and focused person than I was before the operation. True, I was given no choice but to go through with the surgery as scary as it was, but how I fought to get through each moment of the surgery and the long recovery was my decision. I don't think I'll ever lose this fierce resolve which has remained with me, supporting me in every challenge I encounter.

I also gained self-confidence. As each day passes, I feel better and better about myself. Even doing things I'd once taken for granted (like eating solid food) make me feel as though I have won a major victory.

The biggest boost, however, was looking back on the entire experience and realizing what I had accomplished when life threw me an unexpected curve. I had no way of knowing how strong I was until I was tested. Although my long scar and frightening experience may seem like unwanted baggage to many, it has in fact lightened my load, and greatly changed the way I view and live my life.

Epilogue

It's been four years since my operation, and looking back, I am amazed at how my life has moved on. In fact, I wasn't held back at all. I was a nationally-ranked squash player, tri-captain of my varsity squash team, and I played varsity tennis for two years. My best friends and I bowled and rode roller coasters. I can't remember it ever being an issue.

But the most important thing to me was (and is) how my friends have supported me after the operation. My back is ancient history to them and does not influence my social life at all. Sure, I have a scar that still runs down my back, but no one seems to notice or care when I swim or wear halter tops. My (former) boyfriend Steve, a cute and smart soccer star, told me my back was never an issue, and I believe him. And the slight curve of my spine is unnoticeable when you look at me in my day-to-day life.

My back does ache if I sit in a really awkward position for long periods of time, and occasionally I can feel the rod. This can get frustrating for me, but considering the alternative of not being able to fix my back, these minor aches are fine by me.

I head to college in the fall to start the next chapter of my life. I will continue to be neither ashamed nor boastful about my experience but instead triumphant. As I face each new challenge, I will try to draw strength and confidence from the knowledge that I fought and conquered major surgery and scoliosis.

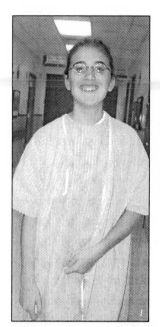
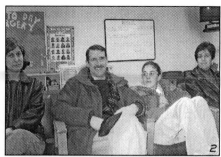
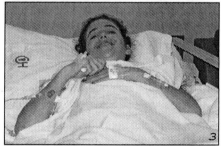
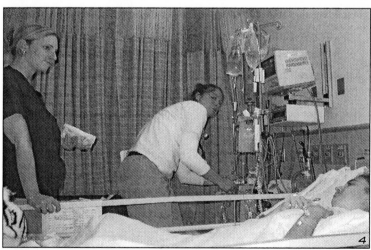

1. Being called for my operation. 2. In the waiting room with Aunt Joanne, Mom and Dad. 3. Relieved that the operation is over. 4. Nurses changing my medication.

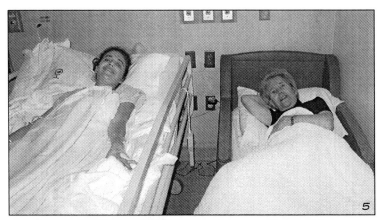

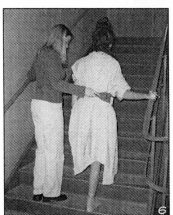

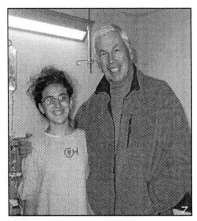

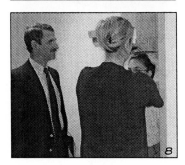

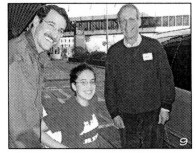

5. Sleepover with Grammy at the hospital. 6. Learning to walk again. 7. With Dr. Drummond on Saturday morning rounds, prior to discharge. 8. I grew 2 inches. 9. Going home.

ABOUT THE AUTHOR

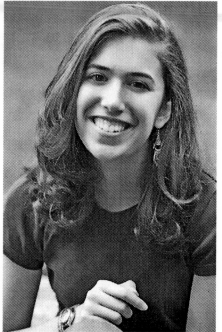

PHOTO: STACEY GRANGER

Elizabeth Golden grew up in Philadelphia, where she lives with her parents and brother. A freshman at Yale, she loves to spend time with her family and friends, read, backpack and play squash and tennis.

CPSIA information can be obtained at www.ICGtesting.com
Printed in the USA
LVOW08s2015240814

400585LV00001B/1/P